Obstet

cket tutor

Obstetrics

Jodi Keane BPhysio (Hons) MBBS (Hons) FRANZCOG
Consultant Obstetrician and Gynaecologist
Monash Health
Assessment Coordinator (Women's Health)
Monash University
Victoria, Australia

Manda Raz MBBS (Hons)
Resident Medical Officer
Monash Health
Victoria, Australia

Shavi Fernando MBBS (Hons) BMedSc (Hons)
FRANZCOG PhD
Consultant Obstetrician and Gynaecologist
Monash Health
Director of Undergraduate Curriculum
(Women's Health)
School of Clinical Sciences
Curriculum and Assessment Lead (Women's Health)
Monash University
Victoria, Australia

JP medical publishers

© 2020 Jaypee Brothers Medical Publishers

Published by Jaypee Brothers Medical Publishers,
4838/24 Ansari Road, New Delhi, India

Tel: +91 (011) 43574357   Fax: +91 (011)43574390

Email: info@jpmedpub.com, jaypee@jaypeebrothers.com
Web: www.jpmedpub.com, www.jaypeebrothers.com

JPM is the imprint of Jaypee Brothers Medical Publishers.

The rights of Jodi Keane, Manda Raz and Shavi Fernando to be identified as the authors of this work have been asserted by them in accordance with the Copyright, Designs and Patents Act 1988.

All rights reserved. No part of this publication may be reproduced, stored or transmitted in any form or by any means, electronic, mechanical, photocopying, recording or otherwise, except as permitted by the UK Copyright, Designs and Patents Act 1988, without the prior permission in writing of the publishers. Permissions may be sought directly from Jaypee Brothers Medical Publishers (P) Ltd. at the address printed above.

All brand names and product names used in this book are trade names, service marks, trademarks or registered trademarks of their respective owners. The publisher is not associated with any product or vendor mentioned in this book.

Medical knowledge and practice change constantly. This book is designed to provide accurate, authoritative information about the subject matter in question. However readers are advised to check the most current information available on procedures included and check information from the manufacturer of each product to be administered, to verify the recommended dose, formula, method and duration of administration, adverse effects and contraindications. It is the responsibility of the practitioner to take all appropriate safety precautions. Neither the publisher nor the authors assume any liability for any injury and/or damage to persons or property arising from or related to use of material in this book.

This book is sold on the understanding that the publisher is not engaged in providing professional medical services. If such advice or services are required, the services of a competent medical professional should be sought.

ISBN: 978-1-909836-74-7

British Library Cataloguing in Publication Data
A catalogue record for this book is available from the British Library

Library of Congress Cataloging in Publication Data
A catalog record for this book is available from the Library of Congress

Development Editor:	Harsha Madan
Editorial Assistant:	Keshav Kumar
Cover Design:	Seema Dogra

Preface

Obstetrics is a unique medical field, encompassing a time of personal significance and vulnerability for the mother in one of the most intimate experiences of her life. Furthermore, the special circumstances posed by caring for two interdependent beings create challenges that are also unique. All of this occurs in a time of wider social change, where care is focusing on shared decision making and adopting a 'women-centered' focus, rather than seeing mothers as 'patients with a disease'.

Pocket Tutor Obstetrics provides a concise but comprehensive guide to the subject. A first principle chapter recaps key anatomy and physiology. Clinical essentials and normal pregnancy chapters cover the relevant history-taking, examination techniques and management options available during pregnancy, while subsequent chapters cover possible complications for the mother and baby. Throughout the book we have included practical tips, clinical images and diagrams to clarify concepts aid your learning.

We hope *Pocket Tutor Obstetrics* provides you with a solid grounding on the journey to becoming a compassionate and competent practitioner. Whether you are a medical student or a junior doctor, *Pocket Tutor Obstetrics* is your portable guide to understanding concepts, passing exams and performing clinical tasks during your obstetrics term.

Jodi Keane, Manda Raz, Shavi Fernando
July 2019

Contents

Preface v
Acknowledgements ix

Chapter 1 First principles
1.1 Maternal anatomy 1
1.2 Prenatal development 11
1.3 Physiological changes during pregnancy 13

Chapter 2 Investigations and clinical techniques
2.1 Assessments in pregnancy 25
2.2 Investigations 30

Chapter 3 Antenatal clinical essentials
3.1 Clinical scenario 46
3.2 Common symptoms during pregnancy 49
3.3 The first antenatal visit 55
3.4 Follow-up antenatal visits 69

Chapter 4 Normal labour
4.1 Stages of normal labour 75
4.2 Intrapartum fetal monitoring 85
4.3 Intrapartum analgesia 85

Chapter 5 Fetal and placental complications during pregnancy
5.1 Clinical scenario 91
5.2 Twin pregnancy 93
5.3 Congenital malformations 101
5.4 Disorders of fetal growth 108
5.5 Malpresentation 121
5.6 Preterm membrane rupture 124
5.7 Preterm labour 127
5.8 Antepartum haemorrhage 131

Chapter 6 Maternal complications during pregnancy

6.1	Clinical scenario	139
6.2	Hypertension and pre-eclampsia	142
6.3	Eclampsia	147
6.4	Diabetes	149
6.5	Chorioamnionitis	154
6.6	Hyperemesis gravidarum	155
6.7	Acute fatty liver of pregnancy	157
6.8	Pulmonary embolism	158
6.9	Other maternal diseases during pregnancy	160

Chapter 7 Monitoring and interventions in labour

7.1	Clinical scenario	165
7.2	Abnormal cardiotocograph	165
7.3	Induction and augmentation of labour	177
7.4	Instrumental delivery	185
7.5	Caesarean section	194

Chapter 8 Complications arising during labour and delivery

8.1	Clinical scenario	198
8.2	Vaginal breech birth	199
8.3	Cord prolapse	204
8.4	Shoulder dystocia	205
8.5	Inverted uterus	208
8.6	Postpartum haemorrhage	210

Chapter 9 Postnatal care

9.1	Clinical scenario	219
9.2	Breastfeeding	221
9.3	Maternal mental health	223
9.4	Postpartum pyrexia and sepsis	226
9.5	Contraception and future pregnancies	235

Index   *237*

Acknowledgements

Thanks to my co-authors, colleagues, trusty laptop, excessive amounts of caffeine and a study door which closes in the face of children's television shows. The book would have been impossible without the support of my phenomenal family, Sir Chas and three patient children, Lily, Gemma and Rosie, to whom I owe more than I can ever express. They are now all in a real book.

JK

Thanks to my co-authors, mentors, colleagues and patients, who inspire me to pursue excellence.

MR

Thanks to my co-authors for their hard work and persistence. Thanks to my wife Sharmayne, daughter Ellara, and son Arlen who have allowed me extra time on top of a busy schedule to complete this book.

SF

The authors jointly thank Tom Banister-Fletcher and Richard Furn for their guidance, patience and for making this book possible, as well as Finland Tan and Aidan Kashyap for their proofreading and invaluable comments. We would also like to thank Lesleigh Baker and Mark Beaves and the Monash Health Fetal Monitoring Unit for providing clinical images.

JK, MR, SF

First principles

chapter 1

A thorough knowledge of female pelvic anatomy, prenatal development and the physiology of pregnancy is required to be able to understand and manage pregnancy and childbirth. During pregnancy, almost all body systems undergo changes. However, these are largely physiological, and many systems return to their former state soon after birth. Other changes, such as striae gravidarum and diastasis of the rectus abdominus muscles remain permanent reminders of the adaptations made by the maternal body.

1.1 Maternal anatomy

The female reproductive system comprises the organs specialised for conceiving and bearing children: the ovaries, fallopian tubes, uterus, cervix and vagina (**Figure 1.1**). These lie within the pelvic cavity and are supported by the muscles, vascular supply and nerves of the anterior abdominal wall and pelvic floor, and the bones to which they attach (**Figure 1.2**).

Layers of the anterior abdominal wall

The anterior abdominal wall is composed of muscles, nerves, vessels and fasciae. It is the site of common incisions made during surgically assisted delivery.

Muscles

The major muscles forming the anterior abdominal wall are grouped into midline and lateral muscles.

Midline muscles These are the rectus abdominis and pyramidalis muscles. Together, they make up over half the anterior abdominal wall.

The rectus abdominis extends from the lower costal cartilages superiorly to the pubic crest inferiorly. It is anchored transversely by attachment to the anterior layer of the rectus fascia at tendinous intersections. These fibrous bands give

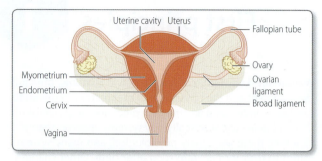

Figure 1.1 The internal structures of the female reproductive system.

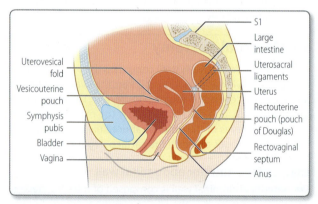

Figure 1.2 The anatomy of the pelvis (sagittal section).

rise to the so-called 'six-pack' appearance of the tensed rectus abdominis. The rectus fascia ends at the anatomical landmark known as the arcuate line, where there is a change in arrangement of the layers forming the anterior abdominal wall; this means that incisions made for a caesarean section do not encounter the posterior rectus sheath because it does not exist below the umbilicus (**Figure 1.3**).

The pyramidalis muscle, which is absent in 20% of people, is anterior to the inferior part of the rectus abdominis and attaches

Maternal anatomy 3

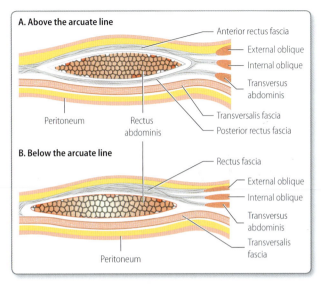

Figure 1.3 Muscles of the anterior abdominal wall, above and below the arcuate line.

to the anterior pubis. The pyramidalis ends in and tenses the linea alba, the thick midline formed by fusion of the two bilateral aponeuroses of the abdominal muscles. The linea alba is wide, superior to the umbilicus, then tapers inferior to it.

Lateral muscles These are the external oblique, internal oblique and transverse abdominis muscles. Their bodies become aponeurotic as they approach the lateral border of the rectus abdominis. These muscles also contribute to the structure of the inguinal ligament.

Nerves

Innervation of the anterior abdominal wall derives from the spinal nerves T7 down to the L1 nerve roots. T7–L1 spinal nerves travel inferiorly and medially, giving rise to lateral and anterior cutaneous nerves that traverse the fibres of the abdominal wall muscles to reach the skin.

Vessels

The anterior abdominal wall is supplied by three sources:
- Intercostal and subcostal arteries (direct branches of the aorta)
- Superior epigastric arteries (terminal branches of the internal thoracic artery)
- Inferior epigastric arteries (terminal branches of the external iliac arteries)

Incisions

During pregnancy, the uterus becomes an abdominal as well as a pelvic organ. Therefore, it becomes accessible via incisions through the anterior abdominal wall.

Pfannenstiel incision This is a slightly curved incision made above the pubic hairline during a caesarean section (**Figure 1.4**). A Joel-Cohen incision is slightly higher and horizontal. Both are frequently used. At the level of a routine Pfannenstiel's incision, below the arcuate line of the rectus fascia, the following structures are encountered, from superficial to deep:
- Skin
- Superficial fatty (Camper's) fascia
- Superficial membranous (Scarpa's) fascia
- Rectus fascia (the rectus sheath) enclosing the rectus abdominis muscle
- Preperitoneal fat and parietal peritoneum
- The bladder (if it is not empty)

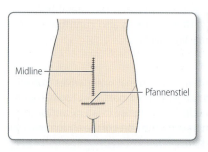

Figure 1.4 Incision sites in obstetric surgery.

Midline incision This incision is made through the linea alba. It is a clean and rapid way to access the abdomen, because of the absence of blood vessels and nerves in the linea alba.

Midline incisions are usually made below the umbilicus. However, when wide abdominal access is required, they are extended above the umbilicus. This is rare in obstetrics and only occasionally encountered during a caesarean hysterectomy.

Laparoscopy incision This is a keyhole incision made to insert a camera or laparoscopic surgical tool into the abdomen, particularly for gynaecological operations. Common laparoscopic incision sites are umbilical, suprapubic and lateral abdominal. Care is needed to avoid damaging any of the peripheral nerves and vessels that cross the area of incision or insertion. Laparoscopy is rarely carried out in pregnant women, as the gravid uterus renders the procedure technically challenging, particularly in the third trimester. When it is performed, clinical examples include for appendicitis in the second trimester.

Bony pelvis

The pelvis comprises four bones: the two os innominata bilaterally and the sacrum and coccyx posteriorly. They are held together by strong ligaments and covered by muscle and fascia. Each os innominatum has three parts: the ilium, located superiorly; the ischium, inferior to the ilium and posterior to the pubis; and the pubis, the most anterior part of the bone.

The pelvic cavity is the space bounded by the bones of the pelvis. It is divided into the greater (false) and lesser (true) pelvises.

Lesser bony pelvis

The lesser pelvis, which contains the bladder and reproductive organs, is the part of the pelvic cavity between the pelvic inlet and the pelvic outlet (**Figure 1.5**).
- The pelvic inlet is the aperture bordered by the superior margin of pubic symphysis (anteriorly), the arcuate line of each ilium (laterally) and the sacral promontory (posteriorly)
- The pelvic outlet is the aperture bordered by the inferior margin of pubic symphysis (anteriorly), the inferior rami of

6 First principles

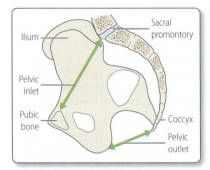

Figure 1.5 Maternal pelvis anatomy. The lesser pelvis lies between the pelvic inlet and the pelvic outlet. The greater pelvis is above the pelvic inlet.

pubis and ischial tuberosities (anterolaterally), the sacrotuberous ligaments (posterolaterally) and the tip of the coccyx (posteriorly)

The pelvic inlet and outlet are the two parts of the lesser bony pelvis most relevant to parturition. During childbirth, the fetus must pass through both apertures, therefore their dimensions determine the ease of delivery.

Greater bony pelvis

The bones of the greater pelvis, situated superior to the pelvic inlet, include the ilium and ala of sacrum. Mobile contents of the abdominal cavity including the small bowel and some large bowel also sit in the greater pelvis. The greater pelvis is bounded by the abdominal wall anteriorly, the L5 or S1 vertebrae posteriorly and the iliac fossae posterolaterally.

> **Guiding principle**
>
> The normal progression of labour depends on the three P's: Passage (through the bony pelvis), Passenger (the fetus) and Power (the force supplied by uterine contractions).

Pelvic dimensions

For an uncomplicated vaginal delivery, the pelvis should ideally be of normal dimensions (**Figure 1.6**). A contracted pelvis increases the risk of caesarean section, however, clinical and radiological pelvimetry does not predict a risk of cephalopelvic disproportion reliably enough for it to

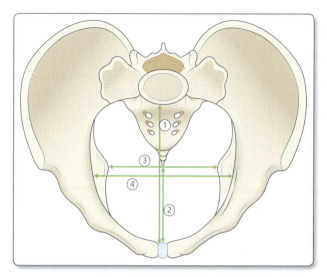

Figure 1.6 Average pelvic measurements: ① Obstetric conjugate: 11 cm; ② Sagittal diameter of pelvic outlet: 9.5 cm; ③ Interspinous distance: 10 cm; ④ Transverse diameter of pelvic inlet: 13.5 cm.

be utilised clinically. The ultimate test of pelvic capacity for birth is labour.

Perineum

The perineum lies inferior to the pelvis. It is bounded by the symphysis pubis anteriorly; the inferior pubic rami, inferior ischial rami and sacrotuberous ligaments laterally; and the coccyx posteriorly.

> **Guiding principle**
>
> Perineal tears sustained during childbirth contribute to postpartum haemorrhage. Successful suturing of these tears depends on knowledge of the layers that constitute the perineum.

Separating the perineum and the pelvis is a muscular and ligamentous diaphragm known as the pelvic floor, which is traversed by the urethra, vagina and rectum (**Figure 1.7**). The principal muscle forming the pelvic floor is the levator ani. This

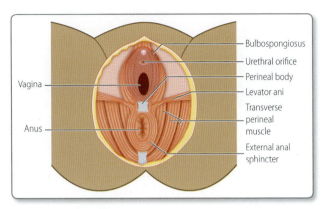

Figure 1.7 Anatomy of the perineum.

thin yet strong muscle helps support the pelvic viscera and is innervated by the pudendal nerve.

The perineum is divided by an imaginary line passing through the ischial tuberosities into a urogenital triangle anteriorly and an anal triangle posteriorly (**Figure 1.8**).

Uterus

Before pregnancy, the uterus measures 8 cm long. This increases to 38 cm by the time a normal pregnancy reaches term, at which stage the uterus lies just under the sternum. The uterus comprises a fundus, two lateral cornua, a body, an isthmus and a cervix (**Figure 1.9**).

Relations

The relations of the uterus are:
- Anteriorly: the uterovesical pouch, separating it from the bladder and loops of the small intestine
- Posteriorly: the rectouterine pouch (of Douglas), separating it from the rectum
- Laterally: the fallopian tubes, ovaries, blood vessels and nerves, all embedded in the broad ligament; the ureters pass lateral to the uterus and inferior to the uterine vessels

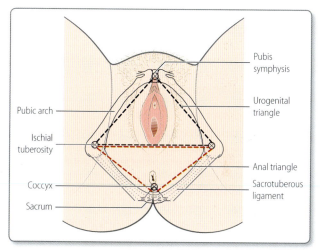

Figure 1.8 The urogenital and anal triangles of the perineum.

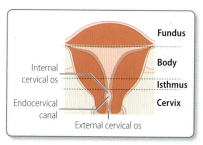

Figure 1.9 Anatomy of the uterus.

The uterus receives blood predominantly from two large uterine arteries, which arise from the internal iliac arteries. The uterine arteries anastomose with terminal branches of the ovarian arteries (direct branches of the aorta).

Placenta

The placenta is a unique organ in that it is present only during pregnancy. Its primary function is to support pregnancy, which it does by:

- Supplying nutrients and antibodies to the fetus
- Exchanging gases between mother and fetus
- Removing waste products from the fetus
- Secreting hormones (human chorionic gonadotrophin for the first 2 months of pregnancy, progesterone, oestrogen and placental lactogen)

Early development and structure

The placenta starts to develop when the syncytiotrophoblast (the outer part of the implanted embryo) erodes through maternal blood vessels to create primordial fetoplacental circulation. As the embryo matures, it develops chorionic villi that invade further into the endometrial tissue lining the uterus until an established organ is formed by 12 weeks of gestation.

The chorionic villi prevent direct mixing of maternal blood with fetal blood and facilitate the active transport and passive diffusion of the required nutrients and gases to the fetus. This minimises the risk of harm from potentially noxious larger molecules circulating in the maternal blood.

The placenta varies in size, weight and basic anatomy. However, it always has two types of surface: fetal and maternal.

Fetoplacental circulation

The fetal surface of the placenta is the site of attachment to the umbilical cord. The cord contains two umbilical arteries (transporting deoxygenated blood from fetus to placenta) and one umbilical vein (transporting oxygenated blood from placenta to fetus) (**Figure 1.10**). At the maternal surface of the placenta, the chorionic villi penetrate the uterine lining, which has become the part of the placenta known as the decidua.

Changes after birth

Once the baby has been born, the umbilical arteries shut down as the newborn starts to breathe. Rhythmic uterine contractions then lead to expulsion of the placenta.

> **Guiding principle**
>
> 'Retained products of conception' is the term for fragments of the placenta or fetal membranes that remain inside the uterine cavity after birth. They may contribute to postpartum haemorrhage and endometritis.

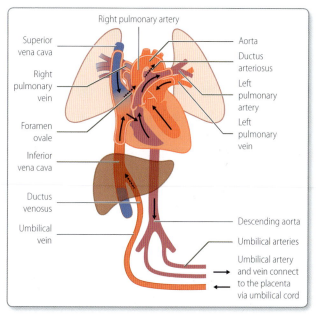

Figure 1.10 The fetoplacental circulation.

1.2 Prenatal development

Prenatal development is divided into two phases.
- **Embryonic:** from fertilisation to the end of week 8
- **Fetal:** from the start of week 9 until birth

Table 1.1 summarises the stages of prenatal development.

Embryonic phase

The embryonic phase is characterised by rapid cell proliferation, by which means the fertilised egg forms a blastocyst. The blastocyst travels from the site of fertilisation, usually the ampulla of the fallopian tube, to the uterine cavity. Once there, it implants in the uterine wall.

Gestational age (weeks)	Events or features
1	Fertilisation → blastocyst formation → implantation
2	Formation of bilaminar embryonic disc
3	Gastrulation leads to formation of trilaminar embryonic disc
4	Neural tube and limb buds appear
5–9	Primordial facial features appear
10	Genitals can be differentiated between the two sexes
12	Oogenesis begins
13–37	Weight gain and continued maturation of organ systems

Table 1.1 Stages of prenatal development

Most of the main body organs start to form in the embryo. The cardiovascular system is the first to develop; the primitive heart tube starts beating at about 21 days after fertilisation. By the end of week 8, the embryo has recognisable external details; facial features, limbs, fingers and toes are all visible.

Fetal phase

The fetal phase is when major growth of organs and systems occurs. The fetus gains weight and becomes gradually ready for life outside the uterus.

Head diameters

The fetal head is pliable, because the sutures that separate the frontal, parietal, occipital and temporal bones have yet to fuse (**Figure 1.11a**). This allows a degree of flexibility, which facilitates passage of the fetal head through the maternal pelvis. If the fetal head is fully flexed at labour, it presents at its smallest (optimal) diameter (**Table 1.2** and **Figure 1.11b**). Presentation of a larger diameter can cause prolonged labour and necessitate an assisted delivery.

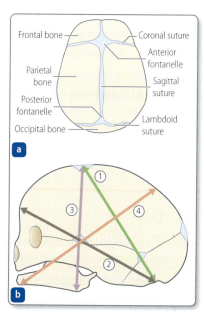

Figure 1.11 The fetal skull (a) and the fetal head diameters (b). ① Suboccipitobregmatic, ② suboccipital frontal, ③ submentobregmatic, ④ mentovertical.

Presenting diameter	Presentation	Diameter (cm)
Mentovertical	Brow	13.5
Suboccipitofrontal	Deflexed vertex	12.5
Submentobregmatic	Face	9.5
Suboccipitobregmatic	Fully flexed vertex	9.5

Table 1.2 Fetal head diameters presenting at labour

1.3 Physiological changes during pregnancy

During pregnancy, the mother's body undergoes various changes to cope with the increased physiological demands of pregnancy. Various physiological changes that occur in pregnancy would be abnormal in a woman who is not pregnant.

The normal values of selected physiological variables during pregnancy are compared against those in non-pregnant women in **Table 1.3**.

Cardiovascular changes

The cardiovascular system undergoes major changes to accommodate the needs of the growing fetus. These changes maintain the pregnancy and facilitate parturition without harming the mother.

Normal findings on examination

Pregnancy results in a hyperdynamic circulation (circulatory volume is increased). This occasionally produces a sinus tachycardia, a bounding or collapsing pulse, a loud first heart sound, an ejection systolic murmur (in up to 90% of women) or a third heart sound. Occasionally, ventricular ectopic beats are present. Peripheral oedema due to vena cava compression,

Variable	Normal range in non-pregnant women	Normal range in pregnancy
Haemoglobin (g/L)	120–150	100–150
Mean corpuscular volume (fL)	80–90	80–99
Antithrombin (%)	70–130	80–115
Alkaline phosphatase (units/L)	30–95	40–220
Alanine aminotransferase (units/L)	7–40	2–30
Aspartate aminotransferase (units/L)	10–35	2–30
Albumin (g/L)	40–50	25–45
Urea (mmol/L)	2.5–6.7	1.1–6.7
Creatinine (µmol/L)	79–118	35.4–79.6
Cardiac output (L/min)	4.5–6.5	5.5–9.5

Table 1.3 Normal ranges of selected physiological variables during pregnancy

venous stasis and low serum albumin is also a common finding in a normal pregnancy.

ECGs in pregnancy

Owing to the physiological changes in pregnancy, the electrocardiogram of a pregnant woman often shows the following features, which are abnormal in a non-pregnant woman.
- Left axis deviation
- Atrial and ventricular ectopic beats
- Small Q wave and inverted T in lead III
- ST depression
- T-wave inversion in inferior and lateral leads

> **Guiding principle**
>
> When a pregnant woman is supine, her cardiac output is reduced by 25%. Therefore, to prevent compression of the inferior vena cava and maintain venous return to the heart, pregnant women are advised to assume a left lateral position when lying down.

Antenatal changes

During pregnancy, blood pressure declines steadily until 22 weeks. It then starts to increase slowly until it reaches pre-pregnancy levels at term. To meet the increased oxygen delivery requirements in pregnancy, stroke volume and heart rate increase (the latter by 10–20 beats per minute) (**Figure 1.12**).

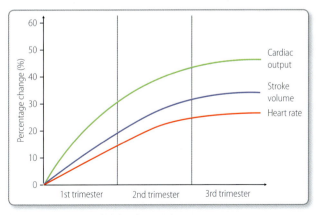

Figure 1.12 Physiological cardiac changes during pregnancy.

Thus, cardiac output increases by up to 40% during pregnancy; half of this increase occurs by 8 weeks of gestation. Maximal cardiac output is reached at 28 weeks.

Concurrently, systemic vasodilation in response to an oestrogen-dependent increase in production of vasodilatory substances leads to a 25–30% decrease in systemic vascular resistance. However, central venous pressure remains stable.

Compression of the major veins in the pelvis by the enlarged uterus reduces venous return. This effect contributes to the development of varicose veins and pedal oedema.

The relative haemodilution that occurs in pregnancy reduces colloid osmotic pressure by 10–15%. This helps explain why pregnant women are at higher risk of acute pulmonary oedema.

Intrapartum changes

Cardiac output increases by 15% during the first stage of labour and by up to 50% in the second stage. In addition, during each contraction, 300–500 mL of blood is autotransfused from the uterus into the maternal circulation.

Postpartum changes

Because of relief of compression of the inferior vena cava and the autotransfusion of blood, cardiac output increases by 60–80% before declining rapidly to prelabour levels by 1 hour after birth. During this stage, blood pressure decreases. Over subsequent days, an increase in fluid transfer from the extravascular space reduces peripheral oedema and increases venous return and stroke volume. After 2 weeks, cardiac output returns to pre-pregnancy levels.

> **Guiding principle**
>
> Because of the associated increases in cardiac output, women with cardiac conditions such as valvular heart disease are at greatest risk of cardiac failure and acute pulmonary oedema during the second stage of labour and immediately after birth.

Endocrine changes

Pregnancy-related changes to the endocrine system include major changes in thyroid function and regulation of blood glucose. The endocrine system also undergoes significant changes to enable lactation.

Thyroid hormones

Pregnancy increases the hepatic synthesis of thyroxine-binding globulin. This results in an increase in circulating thyroxine (T4) and tri-iodothyronine (T3).

Beta-human chorionic gonadotrophin (β-hCG), produced by the placenta, is similar in structure to thyroid-stimulating hormone (TSH). Therefore, it has some TSH-like activity, which increases free T4 and decreases TSH. These effects are especially evident in the first trimester, when β-hCG levels are at their maximum. In the third trimester, TSH increases, which results in a decrease in T4 and T3.

Changes in the levels of thyroid hormones throughout pregnancy are summarised in **Figure 1.13**.

During pregnancy, transport of iodine across the placenta increases to support fetal development, and maternal urinary excretion of iodine increases secondary to an increase in glomerular filtration rate. The consequent decrease in maternal serum iodine concentration is partly offset by an increase in thyroid iodine uptake.

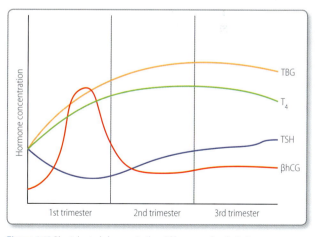

Figure 1.13 Physiological changes in thyroid hormone levels during pregnancy. B-hCG, beta-human chorionic gonadotrophin; T4, thyroxine; TBG, thyroxine-binding globulin; TSH, thyroid-stimulating hormone.

Glucose

Pregnancy is a time of physiological impaired glucose tolerance and increased insulin resistance. These are due to an increase in placental release of human placental lactogen, cortisol and glucagon.

To meet the demands of pregnancy, insulin secretion must double from the first to the third trimester. Failure of this increase in insulin secretion to compensate for the increase in insulin resistance results in gestational diabetes. Glycosuria is a physiological consequence of pregnancy and does not predict gestational diabetes.

Human placental lactogen speeds up lipolysis to ensure that plenty of fatty acids are available to the mother while amino acids and glucose are reserved for the fetus. This effect predisposes pregnant women to episodes of ketosis.

> **Clinical insight**
>
> Sheehan's syndrome is postpartum hypopituitarism caused by severe peripartum blood loss and consequent reduction in blood supply to the enlarged pituitary gland.

Pituitary hormones

The pituitary gland enlarges throughout pregnancy to meet the increased demand for prolactin, TSH, luteinising hormone, adrenocorticotrophin and thyrotrophin.

Lactation

Throughout pregnancy, the breasts are prepared for lactation by the effects of a multitude of hormones released from the placenta, the pituitary gland and the adrenal glands. Two acute events trigger lactation:
- The immediate decrease in placental oestrogen on giving birth
- The secretion of prolactin and oxytocin from the pituitary gland, stimulated by suckling

Suckling This action induces mechanoreceptors located in the nipples to send sensory impulses to the hypothalamus. These act as a signal to inhibit synthesis of dopamine. Dopamine has antiprolactin effects, which decrease the production of milk by the breasts. Therefore, the reduction in dopamine increases milk production (**Figure 1.14**).

Suckling also sends impulses to the posterior lobe of the pituitary gland to stimulate the release of oxytocin. Oxytocin causes the smooth muscles of the mammary acini to contract, thereby facilitating milk secretion.

Urological changes

A higher volume and more dynamic circulation, together with more efficient blood processing and metabolism, improve overall renal function during pregnancy. The increase in abdominal pressure in pregnancy, combined with changes in maternal hormones, lead to higher urine production and smaller functional bladder capacity, causing urinary frequency.

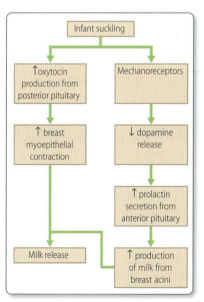

Figure 1.14 The physiology of lactation.

Renal function

Blood flow to the kidneys increases by up to 80% by the third trimester, causing both organs to enlarge. Increased creatinine clearance underlies the normal decreases in serum concentrations of creatinine and urea in pregnancy. There is also a normal increase in urinary protein excretion.

The kidneys become less capable of excreting sodium and water, resulting in increased oedema and salt retention. The kidneys also increase their secretion of vitamin D, erythropoietin and renin.

Progestogenic effects and compression of the ureters by the uterus cause significant ureteric and pelvicalyceal dilatation, particularly on the right side. Pelvicalyceal dilatation of up to 1.5 cm is normal in pregnancy.

> **Clinical insight**
>
> The enlargement of the kidneys and expansion of the bladder during pregnancy can lead to urinary stasis and subsequent growth of bacteria in the urine. If the resultant bacteriuria is asymptomatic and therefore untreated, it increases the risk of pyelonephritis. This is a serious infection that risks miscarriage or preterm delivery.

> **Clinical insight**
>
> Haemorrhoids develop during pregnancy for several reasons: increased intra-abdominal pressure, decreased peristalsis in the intestine, decreased venous return and changing absorption patterns in the alimentary canal.

Bladder function

The pressure exerted by the gravid uterus on the pelvic floor (the main structure supporting the pelvic organs), coupled with increased urine production, causes urinary urgency. This is a normal physiological change that resolves shortly after birth. However, if the pelvic floor has already been weakened by multiple pregnancies and vaginal deliveries, surgery or radiation therapy, stress incontinence or even prolapse of the pelvic organs may occur.

Gastrointestinal changes

Pregnancy causes changes to the gastrointestinal system. These include effects on the gastric, hepatobiliary and colonic systems.

Gastro-oesophageal and bowel changes

Progesterone reduces the tone of the oesophageal sphincter. This, combined with increased intra-abdominal pressure from the enlarging uterus, increases the likelihood of gastro-oesophageal reflux, nausea and vomiting. Symptoms are compounded by the physiological decrease in peristalsis and gastric emptying. The reduction in peristalsis extends all the way to the bowel, causing constipation; and the gallbladder, making the development of gallstones more likely.

Hepatobiliary changes

Serum albumin concentration decreases by 40% due to haemodilution and increased renal excretion of protein. Hepatic release of fibrinogen and thyroxine-binding globulin increases. Placental production of alkaline phosphatase increases its serum concentration significantly as pregnancy progresses. Levels of alanine aminotransferase and aspartate aminotransferase are reduced in pregnancy.

Respiratory changes

To meet the high demand for oxygen during pregnancy, respiratory rate, minute ventilation and tidal volume increase. These changes lead to a minor degree of respiratory alkalosis. Functional residual capacity decreases due to the pressure exerted by the uterus on the diaphragm and compression of the lungs (**Figure 1.15**).

> **Clinical insight**
>
> Dyspnoea is more common during pregnancy, because the mother is more sensitive to CO_2. This mechanism protects both mother and fetus from hypoxia.

Haematological changes

Some variables of a full blood examination increase, whereas others decrease. Haematocrit, haemoglobin concentration, platelet count and concentrations of the anticoagulants antithrombin and protein S decrease. Total blood volume and plasma volume increase by at least 50%. The mean corpuscular volume of red blood cells also increases, and there are higher

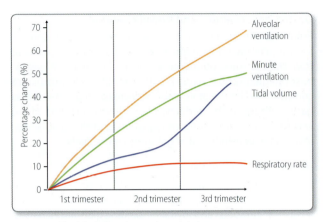

Figure 1.15 Physiological respiratory changes during pregnancy.

levels of many coagulation factors. These changes explain the increased demand for iron and higher likelihood of developing clotting disorders during pregnancy.

Musculoskeletal changes

Pregnancy and subsequent breastfeeding cause a reversible case of bone density loss. However, this is not associated with developing osteoporosis in later life. The effects of relaxin (a hormone secreted during pregnancy), coupled with the weight of the developing fetus, lead to a noticeable degree of kyphosis in the thoracic spine and lordosis in the lumbar spine. There is also laxity of other joints in the body.

Integumentary changes

Pregnant women commonly develop melasma, a skin condition characterised by changes in pigmentation over the face. This is referred to as the mask of pregnancy and tends to disappear gradually after delivery. Another common sign of pregnancy is darkening of the linea alba of the lower abdomen to form the linea nigra. Other changes include stretch marks (striae gravidarum) on the trunk, which are due to its expansion by the gravid uterus, and the appearance of spider naevi (vascular telangiectasia).

Immunological changes

Pregnancy does not lead to a state of immune deficiency. However, compared with non-pregnant women, pregnant women are at higher risk of severe morbidity and mortality from certain infections.

Investigations and clinical techniques

chapter 2

Obstetric history taking, examination and investigation combines general medical and surgical assessment with targeted gynaecological and obstetric appraisal. Establishing the cause of a clinical problem allows formulation of the optimal management plan. This chapter outlines the assessments and investigations that form the building blocks used throughout antenatal care; their applications during the first antenatal (booking) visit and in routine follow-up visits are described in Chapter 4.

> **Guiding principle**
>
> Ensure all tests are recorded in a woman's medical record: results already received, results awaited and any tests that have been requested but not yet done. This gives everyone access to key information at all times; e.g. the notes will show there is suspicion of urinary tract infection even during the several days it takes to get a test's results.

2.1 Assessments in pregnancy

Antenatally, the well-being of the mother and fetus are regularly assessed to ensure that no complications of pregnancy are developing.

Fetal heart rate

The fetal heart is auscultated at each antenatal visit from 20 weeks. A Pinard stethoscope or handheld Doppler fetal monitor is placed where the fetal back is palpable as a smooth line (this is where the great vessels are found).

Fetal heart rate is normally between 110 and 160 beats per minute. It starts at the upper end of the range and decreases as the pregnancy proceeds. Rates outside the normal range require cardiotocographic assessment (see page 40). After 28 weeks, a cardiotocograph (CTG) is also required in the presence of reduced fetal movements even when accompanied by a normal Doppler heart rate, because auscultation provides no useful information for the assessment of heart rate variability or accelerations.

Symphysis-fundal height

This is the measurement from the pubic symphysis to the top of the fundus (**Figure 2.1**). It represents the size of the uterus and gives a rough indication of fetal growth. Examiner bias is reduced by applying the tape measure with the side marking the centimetres turned downwards.

> **Clinical insight**
>
> When carrying out abdominal palpation or any other potentially painful examination, always observe the woman's face for any grimacing. If she is in any discomfort, pause the examination, ask her permission to continue and assure her that she can ask you to stop at any time.

Symphysis-fundal height increases as pregnancy advances. The uterus is felt in the abdomen at about 12 weeks' gestation. It reaches the level of the umbilicus at week 20. In week 38, the uterus touches the lower end of the sternum.

Fetal lie

The fetal lie is the alignment of the fetal spine with the mother's spine. Most fetuses have a longitudinal (straight up or down) lie. Leopold's manoeuvres (**Figure 2.2**) establish lie and presentation. The three descriptions of fetal lie are:

- **Longitudinal:** the fetal and maternal spines are vertically aligned
- **Transverse:** the fetal spine is at right angles to the maternal spine
- **Oblique:** the fetal spine is deviated from the maternal spine obliquely, causing one end of the fetus to lie in the right or left iliac fossa

> **Clinical insight**
>
> From 20 weeks' gestation, the measurement of the symphysis-fundal height in centimetres should equal the number of weeks' gestation plus or minus 2 weeks. Cases of small or static symphysis-fundal height, or a clinically small fetus on palpation, are referred for biometry, which allows for more accurate assessment of fetal growth.

Fetal presentation

The fetal presentation describes which part of the fetus occupies the lower portion of the uterus; this will be the first part that 'presents' on delivery (the 'presenting part'). The three types of presentation are:

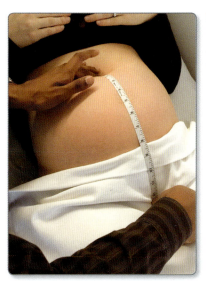

Figure 2.1 Measurement of symphysis-fundal height (the measurement from the pubic symphysis to the top of the fundus).

- **Cephalic:** the fetal head is the presenting part (this is the optimal position for vaginal delivery)
- **Breech:** the buttocks of the fetus are the presenting part (see page 199)
- **Others:** including cord (funic presentation), limb, compound (where multiple fetal parts present together) and shoulder (vaginal delivery is not possible in these cases)

Estimating engagement

Engagement of the presenting part of the fetus is assessed abdominally and expressed in terms of finger breadths above the pelvic inlet (brim). Each finger breadth marks one-fifth. When no part of the presenting part is in the pelvic inlet,

Clinical insight

Palpation of the fetal head to estimate engagement is often uncomfortable for the woman, and it is difficult to carry out if her abdominal muscles are tense. To aid relaxation, ask her to breathe in then out slowly, or to rest her thighs on a small rolled towel.

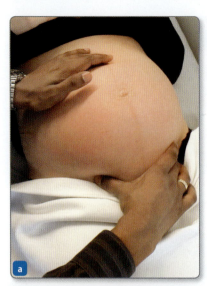

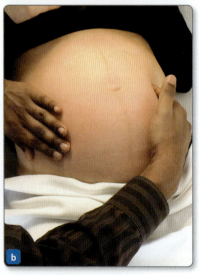

Figure 2.2 Leopold's manoeuvres to assess fetal lie. (a) Pawlik grip; (b) Identifying the fetal back.

this is recorded as 'five-fifths palpable above the pelvic brim'. In these cases, the part is usually mobile, readily displaceable laterally with gentle pressure.

An engaged fetal head has fewer than three-fifths palpable above the pelvic inlet and is fixed. If it seems to the examiner that the head is engaged but it can be displaced laterally, this is a mutually exclusive scenario and they should check again.

Bishop's score

Bishop's score is used to determine whether cervical 'ripening' (softening and dilation of the cervix) is required before labour is induced (see page 178). It is calculated by summing points for dilation, cervical length, station, position and consistency (**Table 2.1**).

Speculum examination

Speculum examination is carried out in the late second and third trimesters to assess for vaginal bleeding or fluid loss as well as for cervical dilatation in the presence of these. It is typically performed in cases of suspected prelabour rupture of membranes or antepartum haemorrhage.

Variable	Points assigned			
	0	1	2	3
Dilation (cm)	0	1–2	3–4	5+
Length of cervix (cm)	3	2	1	0
Station	–3	–2	–1/0	+1/2
Position	Post	Mid	Anterior	
Consistency	Firm	Medium	Soft	
Total score (dilation + length + station + position + consistency)			/13	

Table 2.1 Calculation of Bishop's score

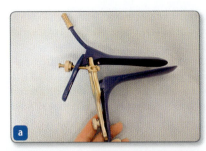
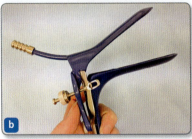

Figure 2.3 Bivalve speculum, in this case a Graves speculum. (a) Closed, but with the vertical opening increased by use of the vertical slide (as for a patulous vagina); (b) Open, by means of pushing down on the lever at the back of the speculum.

An appropriately sized bivalve speculum is selected (**Figure 2.3**). A Graves speculum, a wider type of speculum with its edges curved outwards, is used for multiparous women. The straighter, narrower Pederson speculum is used for vaginally nulliparous women. Sterile technique is necessary.

2.2 Investigations

Routine antenatal investigations are carried out at the first and follow-up visits to identify pre-pregnancy disease or maternal conditions that may affect the pregnancy (**Table 2.2**). They are also used to determine the nature of any pathological conditions, with the results guiding appropriate treatment.

Routine investigations are used to detect fetal disorders. The use of cardiotocography to identify cases of fetal compromise is discussed in chapter 4 (see page 85).

Investigation	Timing	Utility
Blood group, Rhesus status and antibody screen	Booking and at 28 weeks in Rhesus-negative women	Detection and prevention of Rhesus isoimmunisation Identification of irregular red cell antibodies Surveillance for fetal anaemia in isoimmunised women
Full blood count (haemoglobin, mean corpuscular volume, mean corpuscular haemoglobin), ferritin and haemoglobin electrophoresis	Booking	Detection and treatment of anaemia Determination of thalassaemia carrier status
Vitamin D level	Booking, repeated at 28 weeks if low	Identification of need for supplementation to prevent rickets, tetany and hypoplastic tooth enamel
Thyroid function	Booking, and for women with known thyroid disease or risk factors	Identification of need for treatment of maternal thyroid disease, and neonatal screening in at-risk infants
Viral serology for hepatitis B and C, and HIV	Booking, and at 28 weeks for high-risk women (e.g. intravenous drug users)	Identification of need for: • Avoidance of procedures that increase risk of neonatal transmission • Neonatal prophylaxis (hepatitis B, HIV) and follow-up (all) • Household contact screening (hepatitis B) • Treatment for mother after the birth, including cure for hepatitis C
Viral serology for rubella, varicella and syphilis	Booking	In non-immune women (rubella, varicella), identification of need for: • Treatment if exposed • Postpartum vaccination Syphilis: identification of need for treatment with penicillin

Table 2.2 Routine antenatal investigations. *Continues overleaf*

Investigation	Timing	Utility
Chlamydia and gonorrhoea screening in women aged < 25 years or with high-risk behaviours	Booking	Identification of need for prevention of neonatal infection and treatment for maternal health
Diabetes screening, and formal glucose tolerance test if high risk	Booking, repeated at 26 weeks if negative	Detection of pre-pregnancy and gestational diabetes
Midstream urine culture	Booking	Identification and treatment of infection, to reduce risk of ascending infection and maternal pyelonephritis
Dating US	6–8 weeks' gestation	Accurate dating of pregnancy
12-week morphology and aneuploidy screen	11–13 + 6 weeks	Early detection of major malformations and Down's, Edwards' or Patau's syndrome. Dating of pregnancy

Table 2.2 Continued

> **Clinical insight**
>
> Some women decline the offer of aneuploidy or choose selective investigations, e.g. if they have already decided it will not change their approach to the pregnancy or birth. All women who decline aneuploidy screening should discuss their reasoning with a clinician to ensure it is on sound grounds and that their decision is supported.

Blood tests

Blood tests are used to assess the health of the mother and identify conditions that require management or increase the risk of disease in pregnancy. Starting at the first antenatal visit, tests measuring haemoglobin, mean corpuscular volume are essential to identify anaemia and determine the cause. Blood tests also identify cases of vitamin D deficiency, so that supplementation is provided to prevent neonatal tetany and rickets.

Infections

Screening for infections that cause congenital abnormalities or are transmissible to the fetus is offered antenatally. The main such infections are HIV, rubella, varicella, hepatitis and sexually transmitted infections (e.g. chlamydia).

Diabetes

Diabetic women require careful monitoring, because poorly controlled blood glucose levels are associated with fetal growth abnormalities (macrosomia and growth restriction) and complicated delivery (shoulder dystocia) (see page 205). Women with risk factors for pre-existing diabetes are offered screening at the first antenatal visit. If the result is negative, screening is repeated at 26 weeks.

Urine tests

Urinary tract infections and asymptomatic bacteriuria during pregnancy increase the risk of pyelonephritis. Therefore, midstream urine tests (urine culture and sensitivity) are carried out at the first antenatal visit and at any subsequent visits when symptoms are present or in cases of clinical suspicion.

Imaging

Different imaging modalities are used to assess a pregnancy. The most commonly used modality is US; radiography and CT are used to a lesser extent.

Safety

The developing fetus is vulnerable to radiation, especially in the first trimester. This is when organ systems are forming, so major injury is possible. Therefore, imaging modalities that rely on ionising radiation (radiography and CT) are avoided whenever possible during pregnancy. However, no single diagnostic test exceeds the total safe fetal radiation dose, so maternal health should not be compromised by withholding an essential investigation. For example, a CT scan is acceptable if a pregnant woman is suspected of having a life-threatening condition such as pulmonary embolus. The judicious use of radiography is also permissible.

Ultrasound

Ultrasound is a safe imaging modality used during pregnancy for the following indications:

- Establishing accurate gestational age
- Determining plurality (number of fetuses)
- Confirming chorionicity of multiple pregnancies (see page 93)
- Establishing fetal viability
- Diagnosing abnormal pregnancy (ectopic and molar pregnancy)
- Detecting fetal abnormalities, such as anencephaly
- Monitoring fetal well-being and growth (see page 108)

The images obtained are used to help determine if the fetus and its surrounding intrauterine environment are within expected parameters. This would suggest that pregnancy will progress normally.

Ultrasound tests to assess fetal well-being include amniotic fluid index, Doppler assessment and biophysical profile. In fetuses at risk of growth restriction, US assessments of fetal growth are carried out at intervals of at least 2 weeks. With assessments at shorter intervals, any difference in estimated fetal weight is within the margin of error of the test and may not be genuine.

Advantages Ultrasound has many advantages over other imaging modalities. First, it is safe for the fetus and mother, because it relies on sound waves rather than ionising radiation to produce images. Second, US machines are readily available and portable, and therefore easy for clinicians to access.

> **Clinical insight**
>
> The earlier the US dating scan, the more accurate the estimated date of birth. If the pregnancy has not been dated by US in the first trimester, the due date is based on the woman's LMP. This is subsequently revised if the results of the 20-week US scan indicate a discrepancy of over 2 weeks.

> **Clinical insight**
>
> Remember to exclude ruptured membranes, because this also results in low amniotic fluid index (< 5 cm).

Amniotic fluid index The amniotic fluid index is the sum of four US measurements of the deepest vertical pocket of fluid around the fetus in each abdominal quadrant (**Figure 2.4**). The fluid accumulates because of fetal urine production, and the normal amount varies by

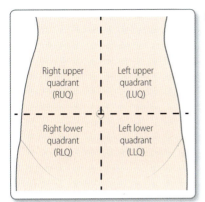

Figure 2.4 Quadrants of the abdomen.

gestation. Renal perfusion and urine output are reduced in cases of placental insufficiency as the fetus redistributes blood flow to vital organs such as the heart and brain.

Doppler assessment Doppler monitors measure blood flow. They are used to assess uterine, placental and fetal circulations, which reflect placental function and fetal response. The four key Doppler studies are:
- Uterine artery
- Umbilical artery
- Middle cerebral artery
- Ductus venosus

Doppler assessment is used mainly for identification of fetal growth disorders (see page 110).

Uterine artery The uterine artery Doppler study is done to assess maternal blood flow to the placenta (via the spiral arteries) and villous development (**Figure 2.5**).

During pregnancy, maternal blood flow increases exponentially as a consequence of dilation and relaxation of the spiral arteries accompanied by reduction in downstream resistance due to development of the placental villi. This process converts a high resistance–low-flow circulation into a low resistance–high-flow circulation. The uterine artery Doppler study identifies any abnormalities.

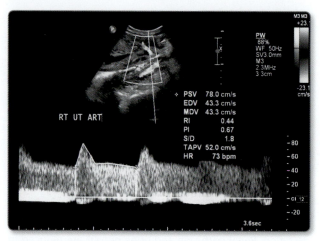

Figure 2.5 Normal uterine artery Doppler.

Umbilical artery The umbilical artery Doppler study measures placental resistance and is taken in a free loop of umbilical cord (**Figure 2.6**). It is most commonly described as a ratio of systolic to diastolic flow, but can also be described using a pulsatility or resistance index. These are used when an SD ratio cannot be calculated, such as in absent or reversed diastolic flow (**Figure 2.7**). The normal state is a low-resistance placenta with high flow during diastole, providing the fetus with adequate oxygenation and nutrition. This is altered growth restriction.

Middle cerebral artery In a middle cerebral artery Doppler study, blood flow to the fetal brain is measured (**Figure 2.8**). The normal state is high resistance in diastole as there is adequate systolic flow. This changes in growth restriction where diastolic flow increases to compensate for placental insufficiency.

Ductus venosus The ductus venosus Doppler study measures blood flow in the right side of the fetal heart and in the fetal liver. Changes occur late in fetal growth restriction and acidosis, and reflect right heart failure.

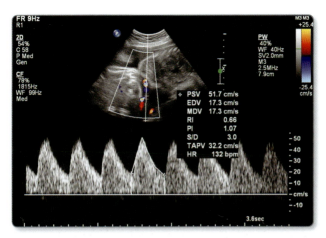

Figure 2.6 Normal umbilical artery Doppler.

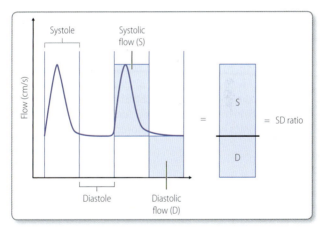

Figure 2.7 Calculating an SD ratio from a normal waveform with positive diastolic flow.

Biophysical profile The biophysical profile is a test of fetal well-being and comprises the results for four US markers and the cardiotocograph. If the US scan is normal, CTG can be omitted, as it does not improve the predictive value of the test. Each

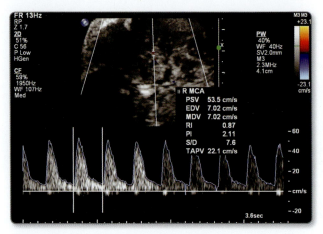

Figure 2.8 Normal middle cerebral artery Doppler. There is a high resistance waveform with minimal diastolic flow, which is normal in this circulation.

marker is assigned a value of 2 if normal and 0 if abnormal. The test may be continued for up to 30 minutes. The maximum possible score is 10/10 with CTG, or 8/8 if CTG is omitted (**Table 2.3**).

A score of 6/10 is equivocal; at or close to term, it prompts delivery. A score of 4/10 is abnormal. With a score of zero, 60% of fetuses will die in the subsequent week, unless they are delivered. Oligohydramnios worsens the prognostic significance, score for score.

The components of the biophysical profile most associated with perinatal mortality within 1 week are absence of fetal movement and overall score.

Aneuploidy screening

Aneuploidy screening is used to estimate the probability of the fetus having a chromosomal abnormality. It is offered to all women, regardless of age-related background risk. The risk of aneuploidy is assessed based on maternal age; information from the medical, obstetric and family histories; and examination findings (e.g. the presence of maternal dysmorphic features).

Component	Normal result (score 2), abnormal result (score 0)
Breathing	One or more 30-second episodes of fetal breathing
Movement	Three or more fetal gross body movements
Tone	One or more episodes of movement from flexion to extension and back or opening and closing of fetal hand
Amniotic fluid index	Deepest pocket ≥ 2 cm
Cardiotocograph	Normal (Figure 2.10)
Total score = breathing + movement + tone + AFI	/8 /10 if cardiotocograph included

Table 2.3 Biophysical profile scoring

There are many types of aneuploidy (see Chapter 5). The three that are screened for antenatally are those compatible with live birth:
- Down syndrome (trisomy 21, see page 101)
- Edwards' syndrome (trisomy 18, see page 102)
- Patau syndrome (trisomy 13, see page 103)

Types of aneuploidy screening

There are different types of aneuploidy screening tests. Non-invasive methods are listed in **Figure 2.9**. If the result raises suspicion of chromosomal abnormality, invasive confirmation testing is offered in the form of chorionic villus sampling or amniocentesis (see page 44).

In first trimester combined screening (at weeks 10–14), maternal serum β-hCG and pregnancy-associated plasma protein A are combined with US measurements of nuchal transparency thickness (fluid at the back of the fetal neck) to calculate likelihood of chromosomal abnormality. This test also gives biochemical information about the risk of an adverse pregnancy outcome, including early-onset pre-eclampsia and fetal growth restriction. Cell-free fetal DNA (also called non-invasive prenatal testing) does not provide information regarding pre-eclampsia risk.

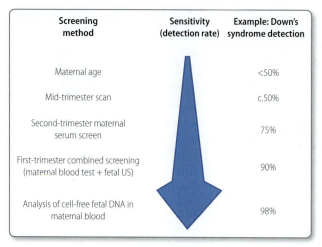

Figure 2.9 Types of aneuploidy screening tests.

Cardiotocography

Cardiotocography records uterine activity and fetal heart rate. It should also include maternal heart rate recording to avoid misinterpretation of the maternal data as fetal. The normal cardiotocograph has two strips, fetal (and maternal) heart rate above and contractions below (**Figure 2.10**).

Interpretation is systematic, following the mnemonic 'Dr-C-BraVADO' (**Table 2.4**). Abnormal findings are discussed on page 165.

Normal cardiotocograph

A normal cardiotocograph must have all features within the normal criteria. A non-reassuring cardiotocograph has one feature outside the criteria. An abnormal cardiotocograph has two or more features outside the criteria or any of the following alone:
- Baseline fetal heart rate ≥170 beats per minute or ≤100 beats per minute

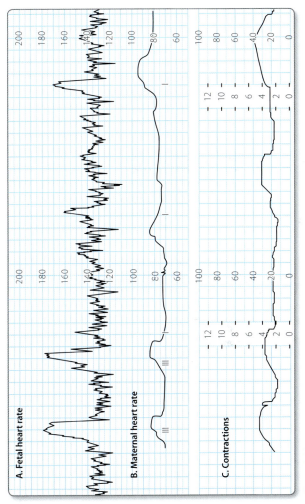

Figure 2.10 Normal cardiotocograph.

Letters	Feature	Interpretation
Dr	Define risk	List risk factors (maternal, fetal and labour) to help assess the significance of the CTG pattern
C	Contractions	Number, length, strength in a 10-minute period (by convention) Three strong contractions lasting 45 seconds in a 10-minute period would be documented as 'CTX 3: 10 strong, 45 seconds'
Bra	Baseline rate	The normal CTG has a baseline of 110–160 beats per minute; this implies normal baroreceptor, chemoreceptor and cardioregulatory centre function and indicates fetal well-being
V	Variability	6–25 beats, taken from the highest point to the lowest point over a 1-minute cycle
A	Accelerations	Two in a 20-minute phase in fetal wake phase is normal outside labour (a 'reactive' CTG) Accelerations may be absent intrapartum, and if all else is reassuring the fetus is well An acceleration is an increase of 15 beats per minute for 15 seconds after 28 weeks
D	Decelerations	Considered abnormal (see page 165)
O	Overall impression	Well fetus, normal CTG Non-reassuring CTG (one abnormal feature) Abnormal CTG (more than one abnormal feature or clear compromise, such as late decelerations)
CTG, cardiotocograph		

Table 2.4 Dr-C-BraVADO: systematic interpretation of a cardiotocograph

- Absent variability
- Sinusoidal pattern
- Presence of complicated variable or late decelerations

A mnemonic for the possible causes of an abnormal cardiotocograph is the four S's: sick, sleep, submature, sedation. The aim is to identify which of these apply.

A normal cardiotocograph indicates that the fetus has a well-perfused cardioregulatory centre in the brain. 'Cycling' is the normal sequential episodes of fetal wake and sleep, which typically average up to 40 minutes. The fetal sleep phase typically manifests as a small elevation in baseline, reduced variability and absence of accelerations; early decelerations may be present, but they are not pathological.

Procedural and operative investigations

Invasive procedural investigations are needed to confirm or rule out a serious condition. The three most commonly used procedures are described below.

Chorionic villus sampling

In chorionic villus sampling (CVS), a sample of the chorionic villi (in the developing placenta) is obtained for the purposes of genetic and histological analyses (**Figure 2.11**). CVS is offered during the first trimester to women whose screening results show that the fetus has a higher likelihood of having a chromosomal abnormality. It is also used to detect some inherited disorders, such as cystic fibrosis and sickle cell anemia. CVS carries a small risk of miscarriage (about 1:100–200).

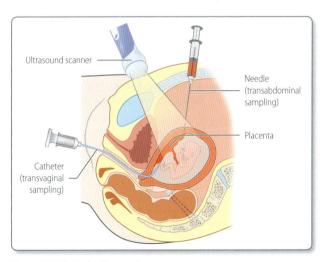

Figure 2.11 Chorionic villus sampling.

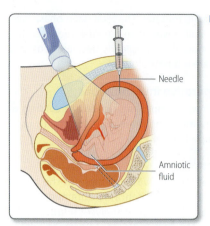

Figure 2.12 Amniocentesis.

Amniocentesis

Amniocentesis is a second-trimester procedure in which a small amount of the amniotic fluid is obtained for analysis via needle aspiration (**Figure 2.12**). This test is offered after 15 weeks' gestation for the same reasons as CVS. It has a slightly lower miscarriage rate (about 1:200–1000).

Fetal blood sampling

Samples of fetal blood are obtained from the umbilical cord in investigations of fetal anemia or infection. This procedure carries a higher risk of adverse effects and miscarriage than CVS and amniocentesis and is not carried out routinely.

Antenatal clinical essentials

chapter 3

The focus of this chapter is the care provided in a healthy pregnancy. Good antenatal care:
- Detects disease or disorder
- Stratifies risk
- Optimises maternal health
- Detects conditions unique to pregnancy (e.g. pre-eclampsia) to enable effective management

Normal pregnancy is characterised by physiological changes that cause many of the symptoms commonly experienced in pregnancy, such as abdominal pain, nausea and back pain. These symptoms require assessment, but they usually cease postpartum and management is therefore conservative.

Modern obstetric care is best conceptualised as an inverted pyramid (**Figure 3.1**): most involvement of healthcare professionals and most decision-making occur in the first trimester (weeks 0–12; **Table 3.1, Figure 3.1**), often at the first antenatal (booking) visit. This contrasts with the traditional approach with its focus on the last trimester, which is still widely practiced.

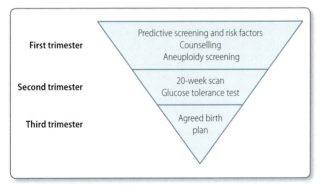

Figure 3.1 The pyramid of antenatal care: the predictive and proactive model.

Trimester	Weeks	Key events in fetal development
First	0–13	All organs start to form
Second	14–27	Nervous system matures Fetus responds to stimuli Hair and nails form
Third	28–40	Body fat laid down Lungs mature (at 39 weeks)

Table 3.1 The trimesters of pregnancy

3.1 Clinical scenario

Nausea and vomiting in the first trimester

Presentation

A 24-year-old childcare worker presents for antenatal care at 8 weeks' gestation. She is distressed by constant nausea and daily vomiting that has worsened over the past 2 weeks. Today, she has been unable to tolerate food but can manage to drink some fluids. Her body mass index is 31 kg/m^2. She smokes 10 cigarettes daily and drinks alcohol socially. No other significant medical or surgical history is noted, and the medication history reveals no use of medications or supplements and no drug allergies. This is her first pregnancy, and she has never had a cervical smear. Her menstrual cycles are generally irregular. She presents with no antenatal investigations to date.

Clinical assessment reveals a nauseated young, obese woman with normal observations. There is no postural drop in blood pressure on standing. Breast, thyroid, and cardiorespiratory examinations are unremarkable. The fundus is impalpable abdominally.

Diagnostic approach

Nausea and vomiting in pregnancy affects over 80% of women in the first trimester, and this is the most likely diagnosis. It classically starts at 6 weeks' gestation, and symptoms ease during the second trimester. Many conditions can cause nausea and vomiting in pregnant women, but in this context, diagnosis is generally straightforward.

Women experiencing nausea and vomiting are asked about features that support the diagnosis of nausea and vomiting in pregnancy. These include typical onset, associated ptyalism (excessive production of saliva), aversions to certain foods and increased sense of smell. Women who describe atypical features of nausea and vomiting in pregnancy are questioned about features of the differential diagnoses, both obstetric and general (**Table 3.2**).

Vomiting that causes weight loss and ketosis and requires admission to hospital is termed as hyperemesis gravidarum (see page 155). It is a rare but serious and often undertreated form of nausea and vomiting in pregnancy.

Further investigations

In most pregnant women, exclusion of other causes of nausea and vomiting requires little investigation. In this case:
- The results of full blood examination, measurement of serum electrolytes, and liver function and thyroid function tests show no evidence of dehydration, infection, biochemical hyperthyroidism or biliary disease
- A pelvic US dating scan shows a live singleton intrauterine gestation, consistent with 8 weeks' gestation, thereby excluding multiple or molar pregnancy
- Midstream urine and routine antenatal blood tests give negative results for serological markers of viral infection, thereby excluding a diagnosis of urinary tract infection or viral hepatitis

Category	Conditions	Features
Obstetric	Molar pregnancy	Fundus larger than expected for dates, vaginal bleeding, passage of vesicular tissue
	Multiple pregnancy	Fundus larger than expected for dates, presence of risk factors for multifetal gestation
General medical	Urinary tract infection, pyelonephritis, hyperthyroidism, diabetic ketoacidosis, peptic ulcer disease, biliary disease and hepatitis, gastroenteritis, mass lesions of the central nervous system, migraine	

Table 3.2 Nausea and vomiting in pregnancy: differential diagnoses

Management

This woman has nausea and vomiting in pregnancy and obesity. Other issues are current substance use, uncertain dating of pregnancy, occupational exposure to potentially teratogenic infections, and lack of antenatal investigations or vitamin supplementation.

She is provided with:
- Reassurance that the nausea and vomiting are self-limiting and unlikely to harm the developing fetus
- Written and verbal information regarding non-pharmacological measures to ease the symptoms, such as eating small, bland meals at regular intervals
- First-line antiemetic medications, including metoclopramide, doxylamine and pyridoxine

> **Clinical insight**
>
> Providing written information is a valuable adjunct to verbal counselling. Along with putting women in touch with support groups, it is part of a multimodal approach to patient education and the promotion of health literacy and independence.

She is asked to return if her symptoms worsen. She is informed about the obstetric complications associated with obesity and encouraged to adopt healthy eating and exercise habits. She is given high-dose folic acid, vitamin D3 (cholecalciferol) and iodine supplements. The importance of hand hygiene is emphasised to minimise the risk of transmission of cytomegalovirus, herpes simplex virus and other teratogens.

> **Guiding principle**
>
> In typical cases of nausea and vomiting in pregnancy, affected women are reassured that the symptoms resolve over time and that the baby will not be harmed by them. In contrast, hyperemesis gravidarum can cause fetal growth restriction and other adverse obstetric and psychological outcomes. Therefore, women affected by this condition require higher-risk pregnancy care.

An estimated date of birth (due date), based on the results of the US scan, is documented in her hand-held maternity record. She is encouraged to stop smoking and drinking alcohol and given details of where she can get support for this.

The offer of non-invasive prenatal testing is accepted. An early 12-week structural scan, along with a mid-trimester (morphology) scan and 26-week glucose tolerance test are also arranged. The nausea and vomiting settle by 16 weeks' gestation, and no further treatment is required.

3.2 Common symptoms during pregnancy

Many pregnant women experience symptoms due to either the physiological adaptations of pregnancy or pathological processes. Although most are minor, all require careful assessment to exclude conditions with potentially serious sequelae. Information gathered from the history (see page 57) and examination (see page 64) enables identification of conditions that require diagnosis, monitoring and treatment.

Abdominal pain

Abdominal pain is the symptom most frequently experienced during pregnancy. Severe pain must be distinguished from mild pain, because each requires a different approach. Symptoms warrant investigation if history and examination suggest a serious non-obstetric cause, such as peptic ulceration, bowel pathology, fracture, cardiac pathology, lung disease or pulmonary embolus, which are uncommon with mild pain alone.

Mild abdominal pain

Benign abdominal discomfort is common. It is due to anatomical, endocrine and ligamentous changes.
- Pressure exerted by the enlarged uterus compresses the nearby small and large bowels as well as the biliary tree, thereby interfering with their function; it also pushes the diaphragm superiorly, altering respiratory mechanics and contributing to the physiological breathlessness that accompanies pregnancy
- The hormonal environment of pregnancy, particularly the increased levels of progesterone, relaxes the smooth muscular wall of intestinal organs, leading to constipation and reflux as a consequence of slow peristalsis

- Ligamentous and soft tissue changes to the pelvis and abdominal wall increase pelvic pain and back pain with movement, due to increased laxity. This effect becomes more marked with successive pregnancies

> **Clinical insight**
>
> **Mild abdominal pain in pregnancy is common.**
>
> Reassure the woman that the symptoms do not indicate a potentially serious condition, and manage conservatively with analgesia, dietary modification, exercise, abdominal support and physiotherapy.

> **Guiding principle**
>
> A 'high index of clinical suspicion' means that a specific condition is strongly suspected based on the presentation, symptoms and signs. It prompts specific investigations to confirm the suspected diagnosis.

> **Clinical insight**
>
> **Nausea and vomiting in pregnancy is common.**
>
> Treat it conservatively, advising women to eat smaller meals at shorter intervals and drink water. However, in cases of dehydration, weight loss or electrolyte derangements, in-patient admission, IV fluid administration, antiemetic therapy and thiamine (vitamin B1) supplementation are appropriate. In very severe cases, which are rare, total parenteral nutrition is necessary to avoid starvation.

Severe abdominal pain

Severe abdominal pain requires a high index of suspicion for an underlying pathology with the potential to cause significant harm. Causes are divided into:
- Obstetric and gynaecological causes in early or late pregnancy (**Tables 3.3** and **3.4**), respectively)
- Other medical and surgical causes (**Table 3.5**)

Pregnancy alters the presentation of some non-obstetric conditions, e.g. appendicitis. Particular suspicion is required, because these conditions have a worse outcome if the diagnosis is missed in pregnancy.

Nausea and vomiting

Nausea and vomiting are common symptoms of pregnancy. The cause is incompletely understood but partly related to the increased levels of beta-human chorionic gonadotrophin (β-hCG) in maternal serum. This probably explains why women with molar or

Cause	Clinical features	Investigations
Miscarriage	Vaginal discharge or bleeding with abdominal pain	Speculum examination, β-hCG concentration and transvaginal US
Ectopic pregnancy	Triad of amenorrhoea, lower abdominal pain and bleeding from the vagina	β-hCG concentration and transvaginal US
Ruptured ovarian cyst	Acute abdominal pain with or without peritonism, hypotension and tachycardia	FBE, inflammatory markers and pelvic US
Ovarian torsion	Acute colicky abdominal pain, nausea, vomiting, and presyncope or syncope (vagal response)	FBE, inflammatory markers and pelvic US
Fibroid degeneration	Localised abdominal pain with nausea and vomiting	FBE, inflammatory markers and pelvic US
Ovarian hyperstimulation syndrome	History of ovarian stimulation (e.g. in IVF) is required. Generalised abdominal pain with distension. Nausea, vomiting, diarrhoea, dyspnoea and peripheral oedema also occur	FBE, UEC, LFT, coagulation profile, midstream urine test and pelvic US

FBE, full blood examination; β-hCG, β-human chorionic gonadotrophin; LFT, liver function test; UEC, urea, electrolytes and creatinine; US, ultrasound.

Table 3.3 Abdominal pain in early pregnancy: causes

multiple pregnancy or carrying a fetus with Down syndrome, which are all conditions associated with higher than expected concentrations of β-hCG, experience more severe nausea and vomiting.

Cause	Clinical features	Investigations
Labour	Regular painful abdominal contractions with progressive cervical changes	CTG or intermittent auscultation of fetal heart
Placental abruption	Constant uterine pain, including between irritable contractions, with or without vaginal bleeding	CTG, FBE, UEC, coagulation studies and blood group and hold (test to determine blood group of mother and prepare for potential transfusion of blood products)
Uterine rupture	Acute abdominal pain with vaginal bleeding and hypovolaemic shock. Uncommon outside labour and requires the presence of a uterine scar	CTG, FBE, UEC, coagulation studies and blood group and hold
Chorioamnionitis	Abdominal pain with fever and offensive vaginal discharge	CTG, FBE, inflammatory markers, MSU, vaginal swab and blood culture
Pre-eclampsia	None, or epigastric abdominal pain with headache, nausea, vomiting or visual disturbances	FBE, UEC, uric acid, urinary protein concentration and assessment of fetal growth and well-being (CTG, US)
Acute fatty liver of pregnancy	Right hypochondrium abdominal pain with jaundice	CTG, FBE, LFT, coagulation panel and hepatitis serology

CTG, cardiotocography; FBE, full blood examination; LFT, liver function test; UEC, urea, electrolytes and creatinine; MSU, mid-stream urine.

Table 3.4 Abdominal pain in late pregnancy: causes

> **Clinical insight**
>
> **Lower back pain is common in pregnancy.**
>
> Non-pharmacological therapy, such as physiotherapy, support belts, and heat or cold pads, is effective for mild lower back pain. Prescribe analgesia for cases of moderate to severe lower back pain, or any back pain associated with sciatica. Avoid non-steroidal anti-inflammatories as they impair fetal renal function and promote premature closure of the fetal ductus arteriosus.

Lower back pain

Lower back pain in pregnancy is caused by a combination of weight gain, hormonal changes, musculoskeletal relaxation and alteration of posture. Lower back pain that radiates to the back of the thigh or is associated with lower limb weakness or paraesthesia indicates nerve root

Cause	Clinical features	Investigation
Gastrointestinal		
Gastro-esophageal reflux disease	Epigastric burning pain after eating or lying down, with water brash and acid taste in mouth	Clinical diagnosis
Gastroenteritis	Generalised abdominal pain with nausea, vomiting and diarrhoea	FBE, UEC, LFT, inflammatory markers and stool analysis
Appendicitis	Periumbilical pain that then localises to the right iliac fossa, with or without peritonism, fever, nausea and vomiting	FBE, UEC, LFT, inflammatory markers and transabdominal US
Bowel obstruction	Colicky, generalised abdominal pain with nausea, vomiting and reduced bowel sounds	FBE, UEC and inflammatory markers
Cholecystitis	Sharp right hypochondrium abdominal pain that is worse with food intake, associated with fever, nausea and vomiting	FBE, LFT, inflammatory markers and abdominal US
Hepatitis	Right hypochondrium abdominal pain with fever, jaundice, nausea and vomiting	Hepatitis screen
Urological		
Urinary tract infection	Suprapubic pain with fever, dysuria, frequency and urgency	UEC, inflammatory markers and urine culture
Pyelonephritis	Loin pain with fever, renal angle tenderness and haematuria	FBE, UEC, inflammatory markers and urine culture
FBE, full blood examination; LFT, liver function test; UEC, urea, electrolytes and creatinine.		

Table 3.5 Abdominal pain: non-obstetric and non-gynaecological causes

impingement (also known as sciatica). Severe pain, especially when accompanied by neurological signs or bladder or bowel dysfunction, is a serious finding that should never be attributed to pregnancy without appropriate investigation. Seek a neurologist's opinion and request an imaging study (i.e. MRI) to rule out a neurosurgical emergency.

Vaginal discharge

Clear or whitish vaginal discharge without offensive smell or associated itchiness or urinary symptoms is physiological in pregnancy. Bloody or mucoid discharge indicates discharge of the cervical mucus plug (operculum) and is commonly referred to as 'show'. It can precede labour by a few days and is non-concerning. Characteristics of vaginal discharge in cases of infection are listed in **Table 3.6**; treatment is required.

Breast fullness and tenderness

Before pregnancy, a woman's breasts are composed mainly of adipose tissue. During pregnancy, the effects of oestrogen, progesterone and prolactin increase glandular breast tissue. This results in an increase in breast fullness and tenderness.

> **Clinical insight**
>
> Watery vaginal discharge is a sign of ruptured membranes. This possibility must be excluded during clinical assessment, particularly before a digital examination (as this procedure increases the risk of infection in the presence of ruptured membranes).

> **Clinical insight**
>
> **Management of carpal tunnel syndrome in pregnancy**
>
> Reduce oedema in the carpal tunnel by elevating the arm during sleep, simple hand exercises and splinting, to allow the nerve to resume normal conduction.

Peripheral oedema

Increased plasma volume, hormonal fluctuations and pressure exerted on the pelvic venous system by the gravid uterus all contribute to leakage of fluid from the intravascular compartment to the interstitial space. This phenomenon manifests as lower limb peripheral oedema. In the absence of other signs of a serious cause, the woman is reassured that the oedema is physiological and will resolve after the birth.

Carpal tunnel syndrome is an example of oedema-related nerve impingement. The median nerve is compressed as it passes through the carpal tunnel on the ventral aspect of the wrist, resulting in

Infection type	Infection	Characteristics
Yeast	Candidiasis (*Candida* spp.)	Thick, cottage cheese-like; accompanied by pruritus
Bacterial	Bacterial vaginosis	Milky white, thin; fishy odour
Sexually transmitted	Chlamydia (*Chlamydia trachomatis*) Gonorrhoea (*Neisseria gonorrhoeae*) Other cervical pathology	Clear and profuse; associated with post-coital bleeding, urinary symptoms
Protozoal	Trichomoniasis (*Trichomonas vaginalis*)	Yellow or grey, frothy; associated with pruritus, dysuria

Table 3.6 Vaginal discharge: types indicating infection

impaired sensory conduction and subsequent palm and finger paraesthesia and pain. These symptoms resolve postpartum.

Sleep disturbance

Disrupted sleep, particularly during late pregnancy, is common. It is caused by a combination of musculoskeletal factors (the altered position of the ribs, hip pain from lying on one side and the need to wake fully to change to the other side), respiratory factors (airway and nasal congestion and disrupted breathing) and frequent urination.

> **Clinical insight**
>
> Do not reassure a pregnant woman that sleep disturbance is her body's way of 'preparing for the new baby'. This is rarely well received! It is more appropriate to gently reassure her that her experience is normal.

3.3 The first antenatal visit

The first antenatal visit, commonly referred to as the booking or booking-in visit, provides the essential information needed to guide subsequent care in pregnancy and childbirth. During this visit:

- A full history is taken
- A general and obstetric examination is performed
- Risk factors are assessed to determine whether a midwifery model of care, a medical model of care or a combination of both is most appropriate, based on the complexity of the pregnancy
- Pregnancy care, including investigations, is planned

The visit takes place as early in the pregnancy as possible, because of the limited window available for aneuploidy screening and the necessity for timely initiation of pre-eclampsia prophylaxis or other preventative interventions. Furthermore, lifestyle and dietary advice is best provided in the early stages of pregnancy, when the embryo is most susceptible to teratogenesis. Ideally, the pregnancy will have been planned and the woman has attended for preconception care. However, at least half of pregnancies are unplanned.

The first visit provides an opportunity to counsel women about normal and abnormal symptoms, healthy lifestyle and normal weight gain, and routine blood tests and other investigations. It is also a chance to answer any questions the woman may have. It should always be kept in mind that pregnancy and childbirth are physiological events and not disease processes, and that the woman should be actively involved in decision-making regarding her care.

Any medical concerns are documented in the woman's

> **Clinical insight**
>
> In obstetrics, the term 'model of care' refers to the approach to providing care for women and babies during pregnancy, at delivery and in the postnatal period. An obstetrician is the lead healthcare professional in higher-risk pregnancies, and a midwife or trained general practitioner in low-risk, uncomplicated pregnancies. In medium-risk pregnancies, the responsibility is shared by a mix of healthcare professionals.

> **Guiding principle**
>
> Information obtained at the first antenatal (booking) visit is used to guide the care a woman and her baby receive during pregnancy, at delivery and in the postnatal period. Therefore, a detailed history and thorough examination are required. The subsequent antenatal care follow-up visits are usually much briefer and focus on ensuring that the pregnancy is progressing healthily.

pregnancy record as a list of issues. This is referred to and updated at each visit.

History

A full history is taken to obtain general medical, surgical, obstetric, gynaecological and other relevant information (see chapter 2). The history is used to identify risk factors for complications in pregnancy, so that these may be anticipated.

Building rapport

A key skill in obstetrics is the ability to establish rapport with the woman being cared for. This is done verbally and non-verbally.
- Verbal rapport is built by addressing the woman by name and summarising out loud what she has said to indicate that you have been listening; this may include repeating the symptoms she has described back to her
- Non-verbal rapport is achieved by using appropriate body language (e.g. shaking hands, nodding and gesturing)

Allow the woman enough time for her to state her concerns, and do not be afraid to listen without interjecting. Women will rarely talk for so long as to delay a consultation. Furthermore, time is often saved if the woman feels that her concerns have been acknowledged and addressed.

The woman has the final say on any decision regarding her pregnancy or birth; however, she may wish to include her partner or support person in consultations.

Age and occupation

Asking the woman's age and occupation is the standard

> **Clinical insight**
>
> The key aims of history taking at the first antenatal visit are:
> - Establish the estimated date of birth and its reliability
> - Clarify known medical problems
> - Minimise exposure to potential teratogens, including alcohol and certain prescribed medications (see page 58)
> - Ensure that the woman is taking a supplement containing the recommended dose of folic acid
> - Guide management to achieve adequate control of minor symptoms such as nausea and vomiting

way to start the history taking. This provides key information for assessing the risk of complications.

Age Age has a significant influence on pregnancy and birth. Increasing maternal age is associated with higher risk of fetal chromosomal abnormalities, medical disorders during pregnancy (e.g. gestational diabetes and pre-eclampsia) and complicated delivery (e.g. caesarean section). Furthermore, older women are more likely to have an underlying medical condition, such as pre-existing hypertension.

Occupation The woman's occupation guides the approach to her care. Some occupations expose workers to teratogenic substances. Others involve strenuous physical duties. Compared with office workers, manual workers in the farming, mining and construction industries are at increased risk of adverse pregnancy outcomes (low birth weight, small-for-gestational-age and preterm delivery). They are also more susceptible to musculoskeletal injuries (endocrine changes make musculoskeletal disorders more common in pregnancy).

A comprehensive pregnancy plan includes appropriate methods to screen for and address occupational risks. Pregnancy alone is not a reason for the woman to cease any physical activity that she is accustomed to and is comfortable continuing.

Current pregnancy

At the first antenatal visit, the gestational age is estimated and the woman's feelings about the pregnancy are ascertained. At follow-up visits, the progress of the pregnancy is monitored and any problems addressed.

Initially, the woman is asked about:
- Her most recent menstrual period and the presence of pregnancy symptoms (e.g. nausea, vomiting and breast fullness)
- Medications she took and potential teratogens she was exposed to around the time of conception [e.g. isotretinoin, anticoagulant or angiotensin-converting enzyme (ACE) inhibitors]
- Vaginal bleeding or lower abdominal pain (these can indicate miscarriage or ectopic pregnancy)

- Pregnancy tests she has taken
- Whether the pregnancy was planned or unplanned, and spontaneous or achieved through assisted reproductive techniques
- The woman's emotional adjustment to the pregnancy (not all pregnancies are welcome)

Medical history

The woman is asked if she has any conditions requiring specialist care or active treatment. These include serious respiratory, cardiac or renal diseases.

Surgical history

Information from the woman's surgical history is used to identify risk factors for complications in pregnancy, birth and intrapartum analgesia. Specific enquiries are made about:
- Spinal surgeries, as these increase the risk of encountering difficulties with neuraxial blockade (epidural and spinal anaesthesia)
- Abdominal surgeries, which may have caused adhesions and distortion of anatomy
- Previous adverse reactions to general anaesthesia (e.g. allergies) or intubation difficulties (due to morbid obesity or a narrow pharynx)

Medication history

The woman is asked about her use of medications and supplements. Specific enquiries are made about the following:
- Pregnancy multivitamins: pregnant women are advised to take 0.5 mg of folic acid, 1000 IU of vitamin D (especially for those with limited sun exposure) and 150 μg of iodine daily
- All medications or supplements taken in the first trimester; these include complementary treatments (e.g. herbal supplements). Type, dose and frequency of administration are all recorded. Certain commonly prescribed medications are contraindicated in pregnancy. Examples include retinoic acid (for acne), ACE inhibitors (for hypertension) and warfarin (for thrombosis)

- Allergies and the nature of the allergic reaction: antibiotics are used both at term for group B streptococci prophylaxis and in cases of preterm labour or preterm prelabour rupture of membranes, and allergies to these medications are common

Obstetric history

Information is gathered about any previous pregnancies, including the number of terminations, miscarriages or live births (and modes of delivery). Note any antenatal, intrapartum or postpartum complications, such as pre-eclampsia, gestational diabetes, preterm birth, growth restriction, postpartum haemorrhage and depression. Pre-eclampsia screening and the use of prophylactic low-dose aspirin are considered for women with increased risk of the condition, including previous pre-eclampsia, positive family history, multiple pregnancy, advanced maternal age and obesity.

Documenting previous pregnancies

Pregnancies are documented in chronological order. Year, place of birth, mode of birth, birth weight and complications are all recorded. A list of G's and P's is generated: Gravida, meaning all pregnancies regardless of outcome, and Parity, meaning all deliveries after 20 weeks' gestation (**Table 3.7**). Multiple pregnancies are denoted by '+' and stillbirth (birth occurring after 20 weeks or birth weight < 500 g) by '−'.

Gynaecological history

The gynaecological history yields information used to determine the estimated date of birth. It can also identify potential causes of cervical insufficiency (the inability of the cervix to retain a pregnancy past the second trimester) and is an opportunity for well-woman care, such as cervical screening.

Menstruation

The date of the first day of the woman's last menstrual period (LMP) is recorded. It is used to estimate the gestational age of the pregnancy and the estimated date of birth ('due date'), usually by means of an electronic application ('app') or a pregnancy wheel.

Situation	Nomenclature
Pregnant, with a history of one miscarriage and a twin birth	G3P1+1: three pregnancies, one birth with one extra baby
Pregnant again, having had a stillbirth at 20 weeks	G2P1-1: two pregnancies, one birth at > 20 weeks and no surviving baby
Pregnant after a miscarriage at 19 weeks	G2P0: two pregnancies, no births at > 20 weeks. Without an addendum stating that the woman is currently pregnant, this could also summarise the situation of a non-pregnant woman who has had two first-trimester miscarriages; therefore, a brief list or description is useful
Pregnant, having had twins then a stillbirth	G3P2+1-1: three pregnancies, two births, one extra baby and one loss at > 20 weeks

Table 3.7 Gravidity and parity: example records of pregnancy history

Regularity

Irregular periods are most commonly associated with polycystic ovarian syndrome. Disorders of the thyroid, adrenal gland and hypothalamus are uncommon causes. Irregular cycles can make it more difficult for a woman to conceive. They also make dating a pregnancy based on LMP less accurate. An early pregnancy US scan to calculate the estimated date of birth is recommended for all pregnancies, but irregular cycles make it mandatory.

> **Clinical insight**
>
> Naegele's rule is used to calculate the estimated date of birth manually: 9 months and 7 days are added to the first day of the last menstrual period (LMP) to give a reasonably accurate due date. The rule does not allow for months with fewer than 31 days, nor does it correct for menstrual cycles shorter or longer than 28 days; therefore, the appropriate number of days needs to be added or subtracted.

Bleeding pattern and duration Normal menstrual bleeding usually lasts between 3 and 5 days. The upper limit of normal blood loss is considered to be 80 mL. However, women rarely measure the volume of their menstrual loss, so heavy bleeding is best regarded as bleeding the woman finds inconvenient or bleeding associated with iron deficiency or anaemia. The woman is questioned about intermenstrual and postcoital bleeding; these are possible signs of cervical disease. Excessive menstrual bleeding causes chronic anaemia, which is treated with an iron-rich diet and oral iron supplementation.

Cervical screening
The woman is asked if she is due for a cervical screening test. This may be a cervical smear (Papanicolaou's test) or a human papillomavirus DNA test, depending on the healthcare system. She is also asked about any abnormal screening results or treatment she has received for cervical dysplasia. Some treatments for dysplasia (particularly cone biopsy, in which a large proportion of the cervix is removed) mechanically weaken the cervix and, therefore, increase the risk of cervical insufficiency.

> **Clinical insight**
>
> Cervical cancer can develop in pregnant women. A cervical screening test is offered if a woman has not had one recently. It is safe in pregnancy.

Sexual history
Previous episodes of sexually transmitted infections and their treatment are recorded. Untreated or chronic sexually transmitted infections lead to adhesions and scarring of the fallopian tubes, uterine and pelvic cavity, which increase the risk of ectopic pregnancy, preterm prelabour rupture of membranes, preterm labour and neonatal infection. Screening for chlamydia and gonorrhoea is offered routinely to women under the age of 25 years.

Enquiries are made about contraception: what types the woman has used, and whether this was in accordance with the manufacturer's instructions. This is useful in determining the accuracy of clinical dating and in assessing the risk of ectopic pregnancy, which is more probable after the failure of progesterone-based contraceptives.

Family history
The family of the woman or the baby's father may have a history of a heritable genetic disorder, such as cystic fibrosis or sickle

cell disease. Consanguinity significantly increases the likelihood of a genetic disorder in the fetus; sensitivity is needed when making enquiries in cases of marriage between cousins or other close blood relatives. Referral to a genetic counsellor is offered if there is an increased risk of a genetic disorder.

Women can inherit a predisposition to other conditions, including diabetes and pre-eclampsia. Many women with gestational diabetes have one or more family members who have had this or another variant of diabetes. Antenatal screening identifies cases of both gestational diabetes and pre-eclampsia (see page 142).

A family history of multiple pregnancies is recorded. Dizygotic twin pregnancies run in some families.

Nutritional and physical health
Regarding diet, the quality of food consumed is far more important than the quantity. Regular exercise should be encouraged as this is beneficial for mother and child. More than half of pregnant women start their pregnancies overweight or obese and gain weight in excess of recommendations (shown in **Table 3.8**). This increases the risk of pregnancy complications, as well as long-term obesity in both mother and child.

Social history
Housing problems, financial insecurity, relationship difficulties and lack of social support have negative effects on the physical and mental health of pregnant women. Women with such issues benefit from referral to a social worker.

Smoking, alcohol consumption and the misuse of drugs or other substances can cause intrauterine growth restriction, structural defects in the fetus and other adverse pregnancy outcomes. They are addressed by non-pharmacological or pharmacological management, or a combination of both. For example, counselling or attendance of support group meetings is beneficial in cases of substance misuse, and nicotine replacement therapy is offered to women who wish to stop smoking.

For women who are physically dependent on a substance, the most appropriate approach is to minimise harm.

Body mass index (kg/m²)	Recommended weight gain (kg)
< 18.5	12.5–18.0
18.5–24.9	11.5–16.0
25.0–29.9	7.0–11.5
> 30	5–9

Table 3.8 Recommended weight gain in pregnancy

> **Guiding principle**
>
> Obstetric examinations often include inspection of intimate areas of the body, such as the vagina and perineum. To ensure that a woman's dignity is maintained during these procedures, other areas of the body remain covered, curtains are closed, and the door to the consultation room is secured (to prevent inadvertent intrusion). To put a woman at ease, the examiner introduces themselves by name and position, obtains consent to examine the woman, then explains what they plan to do and why; they also ask a female chaperone to be present. Furthermore, it is made clear to the woman that she may halt the examination at any time.

Buprenorphine is used to treat opioid dependence in intravenous drug users. Benzodiazepine (which alleviates symptoms of withdrawal) and thiamine supplementation are recommended for the treatment of alcohol misuse.

Examination

The examination has general and obstetric components. The general components focus on the detection of thyroid masses, breast lumps and heart murmurs (which may indicate undetected valvular disease). In addition, lung field auscultation is carried out to check for evidence of respiratory disease. Obstetric components include assessment of fetal growth and position, and estimation of cervical dilation.

General assessment

The examination begins when the woman enters the consultation room. The features to note are summarised by the mnemonic '**ABCD**'.
- **Appearance**: look for the following signs:
  - Pallor, indicating anaemia

- Icterus, indicating jaundice
- Dysmorphic features, indicating a genetic disorder
- Neck goitre, indicating hyper- or hypothyroidism
- Brownish face colour (melasma), usually associated with pregnancy
- Unusual facial appearance, such as moon facies (characteristic of Cushing's syndrome) or the myxoedematous face of hypothyroidism
• **Body habitus**: notice whether or not the woman appears to have normal body mass index (BMI; 18.5–24.9 kg/m^2). Increased BMI is associated with high-risk pregnancy and difficult labour, whereas below-average BMI is associated with fetal growth restriction
• **Cognition**: is the woman oriented or, as a result of severe mental or physical illness, disoriented to time, place and person?
• **Devices or drugs**: does the woman have any medications with her? Is she using any treatment devices or mobilisation aids?

> **Clinical insight**
>
> **The key aims of examination at the first antenatal visit are:**
> - Assessment for signs of thyroid, cardiac or respiratory disease
> - To determine the size of the fundus relative to gestational age; a larger fundus may indicate an incorrect estimated date of birth, a twin pregnancy, or the presence of fibroids; whereas a smaller or impalpable fundus may be due to a missed miscarriage

Vital signs

The vital signs are blood pressure, heart rate, respiratory rate, oxygen saturation and temperature (**Table 3.9**). Of these, blood pressure is the most useful as it will detect hypertension which increases the risk of subsequent pre-eclampsia, and provides a baseline value for later comparison. Maternal blood pressure is taken in a sitting position. This is because measurement in the supine position underestimates blood pressure, particularly in later pregnancy; the gravid uterus compresses the inferior vena cava, thereby reducing filling of the right heart and, in turn, left ventricular output. Increased blood pressure (> 140/90 mmHg) is a sign of pre-eclampsia and requires further investigation.

Vital sign	Normal value in non-pregnant women	Normal value in pregnancy
Blood pressure (mmHg)	120/80	< 140/90
Heart rate (beats per minute)	80–100	90–110
Respiratory rate (breaths per minute)	14–16	16–21
Oxygen saturation (%)	98–100	97–100
Temperature (°C)	36.5–37.5	36.5–37.5

Table 3.9 Vital signs: normal values

> **Clinical insight**
>
> Accurate blood pressure measurements are essential for the diagnosis of hypertension in pregnancy. Measurements are inaccurate if the size of the blood pressure cuff is inappropriate for the individual woman; use of an average-sized cuff overestimates blood pressure for a larger woman and underestimates for a thin woman. Therefore, determine arm circumference and use a correct-sized cuff.

Cardiovascular and respiratory systems

The precordium is auscultated for murmurs, and the lung fields for crepitations and wheeze. A systolic flow murmur due to hyperdynamic circulation (increased circulatory volume) is present in up to 90% of pregnant women, and in the absence of symptoms or clinical history, is unlikely to be significant. All other murmurs require echocardiographic assessment and a specialist opinion.

Abdomen

The examiner places a fully extended hand on the woman's abdomen and uses the palm and plantar surfaces of the fingers to determine the location of the uterine fundus and assess its size and consistency. Uterine size varies by gestation, as shown in **Figure 3.2**. Any surgical scars are noted; all should be accounted for in the clinical history. The abdomen is also examined for organomegaly or masses. The uterine wall and borders are palpated. Irregularities in the wall are usually due to fibroids.

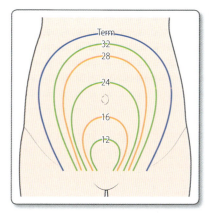

Figure 3.2 Uterine size by gestational week.

Large fibroids are clinically significant, because of the risk of red degeneration (as the fibroid outgrows its blood supply due to hormonal stimulation) or obstruction of fetal engagement (passage of the baby's head into the lesser pelvis) at term.

If intra-abdominal or intra-uterine pathology is suspected, the abdomen is palpated to identify any region of tenderness. Palpation also helps determine the size of the uterus.

> **Clinical insight**
>
> Fetal heart rate is heard most clearly at the anterior fetal shoulder. The sounds of blood flow in the placenta or umbilical cord can be mistaken for those of the fetal heart. They are distinguished by the 'whooshy' nature of placental and umbilical sounds compared with the 'horse's hooves' of the heart. Palpating the mother's radial pulse while determining the fetal heart rate reduces the possibility of error, as does accurate palpation of the fetal lie (the alignment of the fetal and maternal spines).

Symphysis-fundal height (see page 26) is measured from 20 weeks. Between 30 and 39 weeks, fetal lie, presentation and station (the level of the presenting part of the fetus in the maternal pelvis) are determined.

Pelvis

Before examining the pelvis, ensure the woman's privacy is maintained and that any required instruments are available. In the late second and third trimesters, a speculum examination (see page 29) may be required to assess cervical dilatation, vaginal bleeding or discharge. From 40 weeks' gestation, women are offered a vaginal examination and cervical membrane sweep (see page 179) to assess cervical dilatation using Bishop's score and to stimulate labour.

Peripheries

The peripheries are examined for oedema (indicating heart, liver or kidney failure), tattoos (associated with increased risk of HIV or hepatitis infections) and poor skin condition (associated with atopy or autoimmune disorder). On the calves, varicose veins indicate venous insufficiency and tenderness is a sign of deep vein thrombosis.

Investigations

Key investigations carried out at the first visit are outlined in **Table 2.2**. The aim is to detect conditions that change how the pregnancy will be managed or require specific treatment during the pregnancy.

Counselling

All women are counselled regarding:
- The estimated date of birth; however, only 5% of babies are born on their due date, so the woman is reminded that her baby is likely to be born at any time in the range of term (37–42 weeks)
- Minor symptoms of pregnancy and their management; antenatal classes and written information are particularly useful for the primigravida
- The reasons for the antenatal investigations offered, and options in the case of abnormal results
- The proposed model of care
- The planned mode and timing of birth
- Healthy lifestyle: women are advised to avoid smoking, alcohol consumption and certain foods, and information is provided on recommended weight gain (**Table 3.8**)
- Supplementation with folic acid at 0.5 mg/day (5 mg/day for women who are obese, have diabetes, are receiving

antiepileptic medication or have a history of pregnancy affected by neural tube defect), iodine (150 μg/day) and vitamin D (dose titrated based on severity of deficiency), as required

Additional counselling

Details of the type of additional counselling provided depend on the specific condition. However, it always includes discussion of the antenatal, intrapartum and postpartum plans for management and specialist input. Both the effects of the pregnancy on the disease or disorder and the effects of the disease or disorder on the pregnancy are considered.

3.4 Follow-up antenatal visits

Follow-up antenatal visits are shorter than the first. The aim is to check that the pregnancy is progressing healthily, and if it is not, to determine the appropriate monitoring or intervention required. Whenever possible, the visits are arranged for when the results of routine investigations are available, so that they may be discussed with the mother. If any results are missing, the relevant investigations are requested. On average, a pregnant woman can expect to attend between 9 and 12 routine antenatal visits (**Table 3.10**).

History

At these visits, questions are asked about general well-being, common pregnancy symptoms such as back pain and difficulty sleeping (although considered minor, these are often a major source of anxiety) and any concerns she wishes to discuss.

Once regular fetal movements start to be felt by the woman (termed 'quickening' and classically occurring at about 20 weeks), she is asked about them at each consultation. Any decrease in fetal movement requires investigation.

In the third trimester, she is asked about symptoms of pre-eclampsia, such as epigastric or abdominal pain, headache and vision changes, and nausea and vomiting. At term (i.e. from 37 weeks), she is also asked about signs of labour, including contractions, 'show' (discharge of the cervical mucus plug) and

Weeks	Visit	Review
6–12	Booking	All booking investigations (further investigations are requested, if necessary) Usually a consultation with the midwife
14	Aneuploidy	12-week morphology and aneuploidy screen Ensure ongoing pregnancy
20–22	Mid-trimester	Morphology scan
26	Glucose tolerance	Glucose tolerance test Other 26-week blood tests (including full blood examination, iron, vitamin D)
30	Third trimester	Clinical review only, unless other tests requested (e.g. fetal growth surveillance)
34	Third trimester	Clinical review only, unless other tests requested (e.g. fetal growth surveillance)
36	Third trimester	Clinical review only, unless other tests requested (e.g. fetal growth surveillance, group B *Streptococcus* screening*) Confirm fetal lie and presentation
37	Third trimester	Clinical review only, unless other tests requested (e.g. fetal growth surveillance)
38, 39, 40	Third trimester	Clinical review only, unless other tests requested (e.g. fetal growth surveillance)
41	Third trimester	Clinical review only, unless other tests requested Calculation of Bishop's score and post-dates monitoring and plan for induction of labour

*In services that screen for group B *Streptococcus* routinely

Table 3.10 Visit schedule in uncomplicated pregnancies

loss of fluid from the vagina (commonly called 'breaking of the waters' and indicating ruptured membranes).

Examination

Fetal presentation

The examination is carried out to assess for different signs at each stage of pregnancy (see Chapter 2). The accuracy of assessments of fetal lie, presentation and degree of engagement of the presenting part of the fetus becomes more important as the pregnancy draws nearer to or reaches term, when labour is more likely to occur. Non-cephalic presentations need to be identified, because they are not suitable for vaginal birth. In these cases, the options are elective caesarean section in a hospital or, less commonly, planned vaginal breech delivery for a woman who has had multiple pregnancies in a unit with suitable expertise.

> **Guiding principle**
>
> If factors with the potential to complicate intrapartum analgesia are identified, an antenatal anaesthetic assessment is required. This report, prepared by an anaesthetist, is used to guide the intrapartum management plan.

> **Clinical insight**
>
> The likelihood of a breech presentation being detected increases with the number of assessments of fetal presentation throughout the third trimester. Early detection enables timely recourse to external cephalic version (at 36 weeks) or counselling regarding the risks and benefits of caesarean section compared with planned vaginal breech delivery.

Fetal growth assessment
If the baby feels small or the symphysis-fundal height is static or 2 cm or more than 2 cm less than the expected height for gestation, a US assessment of fetal growth is always offered.

Vaginal examination and cervical membrane sweep
From 40 weeks' gestation, women are offered a vaginal examination and cervical membrane sweep (see page 179) to assess cervical dilation and stimulate labour.

Investigations
The investigations required at 26 weeks are:
- Glucose tolerance test
- Full blood examination
- Repeat blood group and antibody screen for rhesus-negative women (to ensure that they are not isoimmunised) before routine anti-D prophylaxis is administered. If they are isoimmunised, anti-D is not indicated and specialised obstetric care is advised.

Fetal monitoring

The growth and well-being of the fetus are most commonly monitored by US and cardiotocograph (CTG) (see Chapter 2). The results of both can be combined with real-time information on fetal breathing, movement and tone to produce a biophysical profile. This includes results for one chronic marker of placental function, the amniotic fluid index (AFI), that reflects fetal renal perfusion and urine production.

The results of regular US scans show any trend over time, e.g. in cases of growth restriction or compromise of fetal well-being (see Chapter 5).

> **Clinical insight**
>
> In some countries, screening for group B *Streptococcus* (GBS) is offered at 35–36 weeks. Women identified as carriers of the bacterium are then treated with antibiotics to prevent neonatal transmission. Antibiotics may also be given based on risk factors alone, e.g. in cases of preterm labour, with similar outcomes in terms of GBS disease. Screening for GBS is not offered routinely in the UK.

Post-dates pregnancy

A post-dates pregnancy (also known as a post-term pregnancy) is a pregnancy that continues past 42 weeks. It is more common in primiparous and obese women. Perinatal mortality is lowest at 38–39 weeks and increases thereafter, and the risk of stillbirth increases after 40 weeks and more steeply beyond that (**Figure 3.3**). Therefore, induction is offered routinely from 41–42 weeks (see page 178).

Management

At antenatal visits after 39–40 weeks, review focuses on signs of impending labour and any maternal concerns regarding fetal movement. After 41 weeks (or following local protocol), a booking is made for the next available induction of labour. Before induction of labour by oxytocin infusion, a vaginal examination is performed to assess whether cervical ripening (softening and dilation of the cervix) is required, using Bishop's score (see page 29; **Table 2.1**). A score of less than 6 is an indication for mechanical (by local application of pressure with a

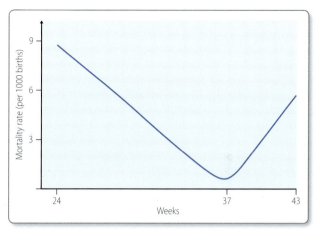

Figure 3.3 Perinatal mortality from 24 weeks' gestation. Most deaths before 37 weeks are due to complications of prematurity, while most deaths after are due to placental insufficiency.

balloon-ripening device) or pharmacological (with prostaglandin gel or inserts) cervical ripening. This process results in prelabour changes to the cervix that increase the chances of a successful vaginal delivery.

Cardiotocography and determination of AFI are arranged for women whose baby has yet to be delivered at 41 weeks to identify fetal heart rate abnormalities or oligohydramnios due to placental insufficiency. All women are advised to attend hospital for review if they have any concerns about the well-being of the baby.

Clinical insight

Induction of labour (when the condition of the cervix is favourable) does not increase the likelihood of caesarean section. At least half of otherwise unexplained antepartum stillbirths are linked to undetected placental insufficiency; therefore, the threshold for offering induction from term is lower than was the case historically.

Normal labour

chapter 4

In normal labour, care aims to facilitate the physiologic birthing process and support the mother in her desired birth experience, while ensuring both the mother and her fetus remain healthy. Emergency intervention is necessary when they do not; this is discussed in Chapters 5 and 6.

4.1 Stages of normal labour

Labour is an active process that begins with a latent phase, progresses to the three stages of active labour, and ends with expulsion of the fetoplacental unit and membranes (**Figure 4.1**).

Rule of three

The rule of three summarises the key components of labour: factors and stages.
- Three key factors:
  - Passage (through the bony pelvis)
  - Passenger (the fetus)
  - Power (the force supplied by uterine contractions)
- Three stages: first, second and third (**Table 4.1**)

Monitoring during labour also has three key components:
- Well-being of the mother
- Well-being of the fetus
- Assessment of the progress

Latent phase

A latent phase of cervical ripening and irregular contractions precedes active labour and lasts several days. The cervix softens, effaces (thins) and starts to dilate. A show (passage of mucus plug) is common. The woman may complain of period-like pain and describe Braxton Hicks contractions of increasing strength.

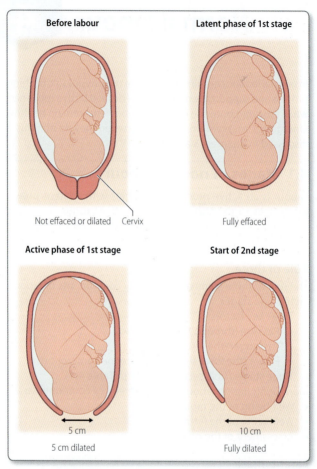

Figure 4.1 Peripartum and intrapartum cervical change.

Braxton hicks contractions

Braxton Hicks contractions are painless, irregular tightenings of the uterus. They are often provoked by activity and do not lead to preterm labour. They resolve with time and conservative measures, such as rest and hydration.

Stage	Events
First	Effacement, dilation, descent
Second	Descent, flexion, rotation
Third	Three signs of placental separation: cord lengthening, fresh show, firm uterus Three components of active management: oxytocic (makes uterus contract and expels placenta), controlled cord traction, cord clamping

Table 4.1 Stages of labour: key events

Urinary tract infection, chorioamnionitis, preterm labour and concealed placental abruption (see Chapter 5) must be excluded before a woman's symptoms are labelled Braxton Hicks contractions.

> **Clinical insight**
>
> Women troubled by Braxton Hicks contractions are reassured that not all contractions represent labour. It can be explained that the uterus is a muscle that increasingly 'practises' for labour as it stretches to accommodate the growing fetus. These practise contractions do not place opening pressure on the cervix.

Management

No healthcare professional needs to be with the woman during the latent stage. However, she can be counselled on how to relieve the pain associated with contractions by means of:
- Immersion in water (e.g. having a warm bath)
- Breathing exercises
- Massage
- Simple analgesia

Advise the woman to call if her symptoms continue without rest or true labour does not commence within 24 hours. If this is the case, she is given a cardiotocography (CTG) and an induction of labour is recommended because a prolonged latent phase is associated with adverse perinatal outcomes.

First stage

The first stage of labour begins when contractions:
- Are regular

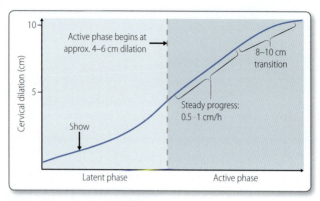

Figure 4.2 Progress of normal labour.

- Are painful
- Last 30–45 seconds
- Occur at a rate of three or more in a 10-minute period

> **Clinical insight**
>
> Ideally, vaginal examinations are performed by the same examiner to minimise interobserver error. This is particularly important in cases of slow progress or suspected dystocia, when inaccuracy may lead to unnecessary or delayed intervention due to incorrect information.

These features generally correspond to a fully effaced cervix that is dilated at least 3–4 cm (**Figure 4.2**). The first stage lasts about 12–14 hours in a woman's first experience of birth, and about 6–8 hours in subsequent pregnancies.

Active first stage

Active labour with steady progress in terms of cervical change starts at 6 cm dilation. After 4–6 cm dilation, an increase of half a centimetre dilation per hour is an acceptable rate of progress. Even then, if the woman and baby are well, patience is warranted in cases of seemingly little progress.

Physiology

Multiple factors stimulate the onset of normal labour, including:
- Stretching of the myometrium (smooth muscle) of the uterus in response to fetal growth

- Peak production of cortisol by the fetus
- Changes in oestrogen and progesterone production by the placenta
- Secretion of oxytocin by the posterior pituitary

Oxytocin acts on receptors in the myometrium. An increase in the number of these receptors throughout pregnancy, coupled with development of gap junctions between myocytes, allows uterine contractions to be coordinated. The contractions spread from the fundus to the lower segment of the uterus, thereby pulling it up.

Inflammation, weakening and rupture of the membranes precedes 15% of normal labours. This is known as prelabour rupture of membranes and itself stimulates the onset of contractions.

Ferguson reflex The pressure exerted by the fetal head on the lower segment of the uterus and the cervix increases the release of oxytocin. This effect, termed as the Ferguson reflex, is reduced or abolished by epidural analgesia.

Management

In the first stage of labour, the woman requires one-on-one care from a midwife at all times, and a vaginal examination is carried out every 4 hours to assess progress. The following are monitored:
- Frequency of contractions (every 30 minutes)
- Pulse rate, blood pressure and temperature (every 4 hours)
- Urine output (if low, this may be because of hypovolaemia or because of compression of the urethra by the fetal head)

Second stage

The second stage starts at full dilation (10 cm) and ends in birth of the baby. Its length varies, but usually lasts about 1–2 hours in a woman's first pregnancy and 5–60 minutes in subsequent ones.

Physiology

The fetal head descends passively until it reaches the pelvic floor. Activation of stretch receptors in the vagina, pelvic floor muscles and perineum stimulates both involuntary and voluntary maternal expulsive efforts to expel the fetus. These cause the fetal head to extend under the pubic arch; the shoulders and rest of the body follow soon after (**Figure 4.3**).

Active expulsive efforts and maternal Valsalva's manoeuvres supplement uterine contractions causing the fetal head to descend to the somatically innervated pelvic floor. If active maternal effort is contraindicated or not possible (e.g. in cases of coma or paralysis), epidural analgesia and instrumental delivery are required.

Management

In the second stage, the baby's head and body are delivered while the accoucheur protects the maternal perineum. A woman may give birth in many positions. The lithotomy position (lying on her back with her legs elevated in stirrups) provides

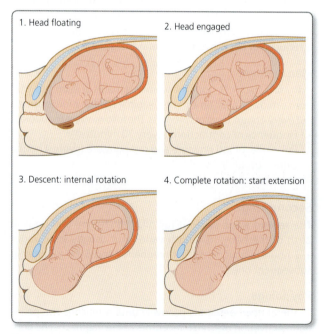

Figure 4.3 The cardinal movements of labour. *Continues opposite.*

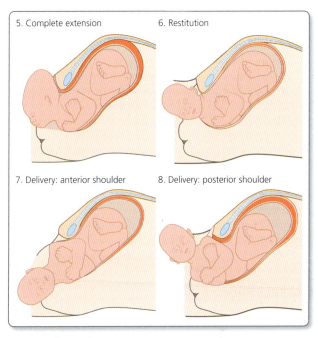

Figure 4.3 *Continued.*

the accoucheur with easy access to the introitus (vaginal opening) and perineum in cases of instrumental birth but is otherwise not required.

Phases of birth in the second stage Normal birth in second stage proceeds in three phases.

1. First, maternal effort ('pushing') is encouraged; the mother is asked to push with each contraction. Warm compresses are applied to soothe the perineum and increase tissue pliability and local circulation

> **Clinical insight**
>
> The person delivering the baby (accoucheur) should always take time to introduce themselves to the woman and her partner or support person. They should explain what is happening and clarify any of the woman's specific birth preferences. Women who feel unsupported or uninvolved in the delivery are at risk of psychological distress in the short and long term.

2. Initially, the fetal head is visible only during each contraction, but eventually it will remain visible between contractions as it descends. The perineal tissue is checked for rigidity, blanching or tearing. If required, local anaesthetic is administered by infiltration and given time to have an effect before an episiotomy (surgical incision of the perineum) is carried out. Episiotomy is not required routinely
3. As the head emerges ('crowns'), the mother is asked to stop her expulsive efforts. The accoucheur uses one hand to protect the fetal head from rapid expulsion and the other to protect the posterior vulva ('guarding' the perineum). These actions distribute the force of the fetal head and enable controlled delivery of the head

Once the head has emerged, the accoucheur waits for it to spontaneously turn to align with the back (restitution; see **Figure 4.4**). Birth of the anterior shoulder is facilitated by angling the head and neck towards the maternal anus (directly down when she is in the lithotomy position but not in others). The posterior shoulder is then born by using the opposite motion, remaining careful to guard the mother's perineum, then the baby is lifted on to the mother's chest.

Cord clamping In normal circumstances, two clamps are applied to the umbilical cord when the mother is ready, unless there is an emergency and the baby needs the attention of a paediatrician on the resuscitaire (an infant warmer and resuscitation unit).

Even in active management of the third stage of

> **Guiding principle**
>
> An accoucheur is a person, usually a doctor or midwife, who assists at a birth. Their role is to work with the mother to ensure that her baby is delivered safely, with due care for maternal tissues, and to attend to her emotional needs. Good technique reduces the risk of severe perineal trauma.

> **Clinical insight**
>
> It is difficult to ask the woman to stop her expulsive efforts as the head emerges. This must be discussed with her before the birth, especially in cases of barriers to communication (e.g. if mother and accoucheur have different first languages).

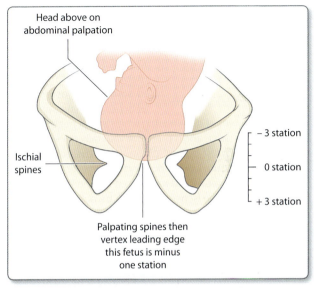

Figure 4.4 Stations of fetal descent. The position of the fetal head is described relative to the ischial spines.

labour, cord clamping is deferred for several minutes or until the cord stops pulsating. This has advantages for the newborn, including higher haematocrit and lower risk of anaemia, but is at the risk of increased neonatal jaundice and the necessity for phototherapy. Preterm babies have the most to gain from delayed cord clamping, as aerating the lungs before clamping the umbilical cord allows a more stable heart

Clinical insight

A uterotonic agent/oxytocic (a drug to stimulate uterine contractions) is administered when the anterior shoulder has been delivered. The resulting strong uterine contractions cause separation and delivery of the placenta.

Guiding principle

Even in urgent circumstances, the woman's partner or support person may wish to feel as involved in the birth as possible. Therefore, they are offered the task of cutting the umbilical cord.

> **Clinical insight**
>
> Always feel abdominally for fetal head palpable above the pelvic inlet (brim). Instrumental delivery cannot proceed if any of the head is palpable above the brim.

rate and faster increase in oxygenation during the neonatal transition.

Key landmarks Bony landmarks are used in labour to standardise assessment between examiners and form a core component of determining when a fetal head has fully engaged in the pelvis and is therefore vaginally deliverable. As part of the narrowest portion of the pelvis, the ischial spines are a key intrapartum landmark; they form a vertical reference marker. Once the fetal head has passed this point, the rest of the baby follows. The ischial spines can be palpated posterolaterally in the maternal vagina and are more pointed than the ischial tuberosities.

Descent of the fetal head is described in terms of the number of centimetres above (minus 1, 2 or 3 or more) or below (plus 1, 2 or 3) the ischial spines, which are termed 'zero station' (**Figure 4.4**).

Third stage

In the third stage of labour, the placenta and membranes are delivered normally with assistance from the accoucheur. Allowing the placenta and membranes to be delivered without assistance from the accoucheur using only spontaneous uterine contractions (termed as a physiological third stage), doubles the risk of postpartum haemorrhage.

Management

To assist in delivery of the placenta, the accoucheur gently pulls on the umbilical cord with one hand while guarding the fundus abdominally with the other hand (to prevent uterine inversion) over several tonic contractions. To reduce the risk of cord avulsion or uterine inversion, this must be done only after signs of separation (cord lengthening, a separation bleed manifesting as a gush of blood, and an elevated globular uterus) and with a contraction.

4.2 Intrapartum fetal monitoring

Intrapartum monitoring is designed to identify and reduce the risk of fetal compromise during labour. The two main options for intrapartum monitoring are intermittent auscultation (IA) and CTG.

Intermittent auscultation

This is carried out by using a handheld Doppler to auscultate the fetal heart both during and for 60 seconds after a contraction and thus detect any late decelerations. It is done about every 5 minutes in the first stage of labour and every 5 minutes in the second stage.

Intermittent auscultation is appropriate for uncomplicated pregnancies. Abnormal findings are an indication to start cardiotocographic monitoring.

Cardiotocography

Intrapartum CTG is a highly sensitive method for detecting cases of fetal compromise due to hypoxia or acidosis. However, its specificity is only 60%, so in many cases, an abnormal cardiotocograph does not mean that the baby is unwell. For this reason, CTG is reserved for higher-risk pregnancies. A normal cardiotocograph (**Figure 2.10**) effectively excludes fetal compromise.

Fetal scalp lactate sampling (where a small sample of fetal blood is taken from a fetal scalp prick) is used to decrease the number of unnecessary interventions, such as caesarean section and instrumental birth, arising from false-positive CTG findings.

4.3 Intrapartum analgesia

Intrapartum analgesia is used by most labouring women. It is provided by either non-pharmacological or pharmacological methods. Differences in the production of pain in the first and second stages of labour mean that a different analgesic approach is required for each.

> **Clinical insight**
>
> Many women feel reluctant to request pain relief, and occasionally there is doubt about whether it should be provided. However, in no other area of medicine is it acceptable to withhold analgesia to a patient who requests it, and this standard also applies in obstetrics.

Production of pain

In the first stage, pain is produced by uterine contractions and distension of the lower segment of the uterus and the cervix. It is conveyed by visceral sensory afferents from T10 to L1 to the paravertebral sympathetic chain, and then enters the spinal cord via dorsal rami at these levels before ascending to higher centres in the spinothalamic tract.

In the second stage, somatic pain arises from distension of the vagina and perineum. This travels via the pudendal nerve to the S2 to S4 dorsal rami, before ascending via the dorsal columns to the higher centres.

Non-pharmacological pain relief

These techniques aim to better inform and empower women to control their own pain during labour. They achieve this through a combination of mental and physical distraction.

The most commonly used non-pharmacological techniques are:
- Birth education
- Breathing exercises
- Continuous support in labour
- Transcutaneous electrical nerve stimulation
- Acupressure
- Sterile water injections
- Hypnobirthing
- Water immersion

They reduce the need for pharmacological pain relief in suitably motivated women who choose them. Education and continuous support are offered to all women, because they decrease fear and anxiety.

Pharmacological pain relief

The use of regional techniques to administer pain-relieving drugs minimises fetal exposure to the medication. Systemic therapies expose the fetus to a variable amount of medication.

Common regional techniques are:
- Local perineal infiltration, used in the second stage for perineal analgesia
- Pudendal block, used to provide perineal analgesia in the second stage and prior to instrumental delivery
- Spinal and epidural anaesthesia possible at any time during labour, as long as the woman is able to sit upright

Commonly used systemic techniques are:
- Inhalational (nitrous oxide and oxygen)
- Intramuscular (morphine or pethidine)
- Intravenous (for opiates, as in patient-controlled analgesia) systemic techniques are usually used in the latent and active first stage

The use of intravenous systemic techniques is uncommon. However, they are useful when epidural anaesthesia is contra-indicated and the woman requires stronger pain relief.

Perineal infiltration

Lidocaine is injected directly, usually to numb the perineum at the site of a planned episiotomy.

Adverse effects The adverse effects of perineal infiltration are minimal. However, intravascular injection must be avoided by always withdrawing the plunger and checking for flashback of blood before injecting.

Pudendal block

This provides perineal anaesthesia by blocking pain afferents from the pudendal nerve. A long needle with a guard is used to infiltrate with local anaesthetic the area of the pudendal nerve medial to the ischial spine.

Adverse effects The adverse effects of pudendal block are minimal. However, care must be taken to avoid accidently injecting the fetus or maternal circulation.

Spinal anaesthesia

To produce spinal anaesthesia, the subarachnoid space is injected by an anaesthetist with a local anaesthetic either with or without an accompanying opiate. The nerve roots are directly bathed in analgesic, thereby providing surgical anaesthesia for up to 3 hours.

Adverse effects These are:
- Hypotension
- Fetal bradycardia
- Shivering
- Urinary retention, necessitating catheterisation
- Need for synthetic oxytocin (e.g. Syntocinon) augmentation due to obliteration of the Ferguson reflex
- Need for instrumental delivery

After the birth, recovery of movement is prompt and a new motor block or severe back pain prompts exclusion of epidural haematoma, because this is a neurosurgical emergency.

Contraindications These are:
- Thrombocytopenia and coagulopathy
- Fixed output cardiac disease and spinal surgery affecting the lumbosacral spine

Epidural anaesthesia

To produce epidural anaesthesia, the epidural space is injected with a local anaesthetic either with or without an accompanying opiate. A catheter is used for infusion and bolus anaesthesia of the sensory nerve roots as they enter the dural space.

Adverse effects The same adverse effects as for spinal anaesthesia.

Nitrous oxide and oxygen

A variable mix of nitrous oxide and oxygen ('gas and air') is inhaled and absorbed via the lungs. It crosses the maternal blood–brain barrier to provide variable analgesia. The full effect is felt about 60 seconds after inhalation and wears off rapidly.

Adverse effects Adverse effects include nausea, vomiting and sedation.

Opiate injection

An intramuscular injection of morphine or pethidine provides systemic anaesthesia. It is given alongside an antiemetic.

Adverse effects These are:
- Nausea
- Vomiting
- Sedation
- Risk of neonatal sedation, peaking 2–4 hours after administration

Fetal and placental complications during pregnancy

chapter 5

Complications can occur at any stage of fetal development. In early pregnancy, a significant problem often leads to loss of the pregnancy (miscarriage) or an ongoing pregnancy affected by fetal abnormality or compromise. In later pregnancy, disorders of fetal growth predominate and the focus is on detection of such conditions to enable appropriate management to reduce the risk of associated poor perinatal outcomes.

Many fetal abnormalities are incompatible with life and some are associated with significant morbidity and require major surgery or long-term medical care. Management of fetal complications is ethically challenging; multidisciplinary input is a must, alongside a non-directive approach to counselling women whose pregnancies are affected.

Continuation of a pregnancy affected by a pregnancy-specific complication may benefit the fetus by allowing more time for it to mature. However, it may place the mother at risk, and if the risk is deemed too great, this option is contraindicated.

5.1 Clinical scenario

A new diagnosis of multiple pregnancy

Presentation

A 27-year-old G2P1 presents 16 weeks into her pregnancy, having received the results of her maternal serum screening test; her increased alpha-fetoprotein (AFP) levels mean that the pregnancy is considered at higher risk of being affected by a neural tube defect. The test was done at 15 weeks, because she missed the window for first-trimester combined screening and declined non-invasive prenatal testing because of the cost (she has not had any US scans to date). She feels that the gestational age based on her last menstrual period is reliable, because her periods are regular and she is certain of the dates of the most recent one.

The pregnancy is planned, and she has been taking periconceptual folic acid at the appropriate dosage. All routine investigations are normal. There is no history of bleeding or other complications. Past medical and surgical history are unremarkable. Family history is negative for spina bifida or other neural tube defects (e.g. anencephaly).

Diagnostic approach

Possible causes for this screening result are:
- Incorrect dating (the most common cause)
- An open neural tube defect (e.g. spina bifida)
- More advanced gestation than expected
- Incorrect maternal data, particularly weight
- Multiple pregnancy
- Several fetal malformations
- Antepartum haemorrhage (in cases of fetomaternal bleeding' where fetal blood which is high in AFP enters the maternal circulation)
- Maternal disease (e.g. liver or ovarian germ cell tumours)

After confirming that maternal weight and other information about the woman are correct, she is referred for US at a tertiary centre (a hospital offering specialist care).

Investigations

The US scan reveals a healthy dichorionic twin pregnancy of the expected gestation. Neither fetus has any sign of a neural tube defect or other morphological abnormality. The placentas appear normal.

The likelihood of neural tube defect is recalculated using the reference range for AFP levels in cases of twin gestation. The new result places the pregnancy in the low-risk category (lower than 1 in 250). The woman is advised that there is now no concern regarding the original result of the maternal serum screening test.

Management

The woman is counselled about her twin pregnancy. She is informed of the increased likelihood of minor symptoms and major complications and the need for medically led care, more frequent antenatal visits and regular US scans to monitor fetal growth. The recommendation to give birth by approximately 38 weeks' gestation is explained.

A mid-trimester (morphology) US scan is arranged for 20 weeks' gestation, and her care is transferred to the twins unit. She is given written information regarding twin pregnancy and the details of local support groups.

5.2 Twin pregnancy

Twin pregnancies are considered high risk. This is because they have a higher risk of every pregnancy complication apart from macrosomia and post-dates delivery. They occur naturally in about 1 in 80 pregnancies. However, the observed incidence is higher due to the use of assisted reproductive techniques and the increased chance of spontaneous multiple ovulations in women of advanced maternal age (>35 years).

Multiple gestations impose higher physiological demands on the mother. They also carry an increased risk of developing pre-eclampsia, gestational diabetes and urinary tract infections. Because of these risks, efforts to reduce the likelihood of multiple pregnancy from the use of assisted reproductive technology include a limit on the number of embryos transferred in IVF (in the UK, two or, in exceptional circumstances, three) and careful control of ovulation induction to ensure that only one or two follicles develop per cycle.

> **Guiding principle**
>
> The 1-in-80 rule also extends to higher-order multiple pregnancies. Triplets occur spontaneously in 1 in 80^2 pregnancies, quadruplets in 1 in 80^3 and so on.

Types

The three main descriptive terms for twin pregnancy are zygosity, chorionicity and amnionicity (**Table 5.1**).
- **Zygosity:** the origin of the twins
  - **Monozygotic:** from one fertilised ovum (identical twins)
  - **Dizygotic:** from two different ova (fraternal twins)
- **Chorionicity:** the number of placentas and whether they are shared by the twins

Fetal and placental complications during pregnancy

Zygosity	Chorionicity and amnionicity	Descriptive terms
Dizygous: arising from two separate fertilised oocytes	Dichorionic diamniotic: each fetus has its own placenta and membranes	DCDA DC/DA DiDi
Monozygous: arising from a single fertilised ovum that splits	Dichorionic diamniotic	DCDA DC/DA DiDi
	Monochorionic diamniotic: sharing one chorion but contained in individual amniotic sacs	MCDA MC/DA MoDi
	Monochorionic monoamniotic: sharing both chorion and amnion and in the same amniotic sac	MCMA MC/MA MoMo
	Conjoined: sharing body components and the same amniotic sac	Conjoined
	Twin reversed arterial perfusion: one of a monochorionic pair dies but the other twin provides enough collateral circulation in reversed fashion through the umbilical arteries to allow continued growth of varying amounts of the lower half of the demised twin's body	TRAP
	One twin develops to a varying extent and is at least partially enveloped inside its twin	Parasitic

Table 5.1 Zygosity, chorionicity, amnionicity and examples of descriptive terms

- **Amnionicity:** the number of amniotic sacs
  - **Monoamniotic:** both fetuses share a sac
  - **Diamniotic:** the fetuses are in separate sacs

Most twins are dizygotic. The incidence of monozygotic twinning is relatively constant, with 3 or 4 births in 1000 producing identical twins.

Day of division	Chorionicity*	Comments	Proportion of monochorionic twins
1–4	DCDA	With early division at the morula stage, each fetus becomes functionally separate and forms its own placenta, chorion and amnion (as in the case of dizygous twinning)	30%
4–8	MCDA	Division at blastocyst stage results in a common placental mass and shared chorion; each fetus develops with its own amniotic sac	About 70%
9–13	MCMA	Division after day 8 results in a shared placenta, chorion and amnion	<1%
14+	Conjoined	Division after day 14 results in shared body parts	<0.1%

*See Table 5.1 for explanation of chorionicity descriptive terms.

Table 5.2 Monozygotic twin types by timing of division

Monozygotic twins These arise when one fertilised ovum divides at an early stage, when it is pluripotent (capable of forming all tissues and organs of the body). The timing of this division determines the chorionicity of monozygotic twins (**Table 5.2**).

The timing of division of the fertilised ovum determines whether monozygotic twins will share a placenta or an amniotic cavity. The earlier the division, the more separate the twins.

Dizygotic twins If two ova are released in a single cycle and both are fertilised, the resulting twins are termed as dizygotic. They have different genetic composition but grow side-by-side as 'womb mates'. Dizygotic twins never share a placenta and, as in singleton pregnancies, each embryo has its own chorion

> **Guiding principle**
>
> Ultrasound is used to determine chorionicity, not zygosity or whether twins are 'identical'. Up to a third of monozygotic twins have the same US appearance as dizygotic twins with two separate sacs and placentas. Therefore, it is prudent not to call the twins in a dichorionic diamniotic pregnancy 'fraternal' unless they are of different sexes are therefore clearly fraternal.

and amnion (the two layers of membrane forming the sac enclosing the embryo). The combined chorion and amnion is visible on a first-trimester US scan as a thick wedge of tissue (the lambda sign). Each dizygotic twin has its own circulatory system.

Chorionicity It is essential to establish chorionicity, because it determines the risks of a twin pregnancy and guides antenatal monitoring, mode of birth and timing of delivery. Monochorionic twins are associated with a higher risk of complications than dichorionic twins. Chorionicity is best ascertained early in the first trimester, when the US signs are clearer. Rare pregnancies, such as suspected monoamniotic pregnancies, require confirmation at 12–14 weeks, because the thin dividing membrane may be missed in earlier scans.

T sign Compared with dichorionic twins, monochorionic twins are separated by a thinner membrane composed of amnion only. This is visualised on US during the first trimester and resembles the letter T (hence the 'T sign').

Rare forms of twinning The following are very rare forms of twinning. These pregnancies are best managed in specialist centres.
- **Conjoined twins:** twins joined at one or more parts of the body
- **Twin reversed arterial perfusion (TRAP):** the torso and lower limbs of a monochorionic twin without a heart or head continue to develop due to reversed perfusion via the umbilical arteries and powered by the circulation of the surviving twin
- **Parasitic twins:** a poorly developed twin, lacking the organs and tissues critical for independent survival, is attached to or embedded in the otherwise normally developing twin

Risks

Compared with singleton pregnancies, twin pregnancies carry about double the risk of every pregnancy complication except macrosomia and post-dates pregnancy (**Tables 5.3** and **5.4**). Therefore, women with twin pregnancies

> ### Guiding principle
>
> Because of the high rates of first-trimester diagnosis and up to 15% likelihood of the loss of one twin in the first trimester due to spontaneous miscarriage, some twin pregnancies continue as a singleton pregnancy. This is called vanishing twin syndrome.

Stage	Minor risks	Major risks
First trimester	Nausea and vomiting Fatigue	Hyperemesis
Second and third trimesters	Back and pelvic pain Reflux More visible striae gravidarum Breathlessness Poor sleep Fatigue Antepartum haemorrhage (minor)	Pre-eclampsia Pregnancy-induced hypertension Gestational diabetes mellitus Placenta praevia, vasa praevia Antepartum haemorrhage (major)
Intrapartum	Increased likelihood of: Induction of labour Synthetic oxytocin (Syntocinon) use Epidural anaesthesia Instrumental delivery Postpartum haemorrhage (minor)	Increased likelihood of caesarean section Postpartum haemorrhage (major)
Postpartum	Breastfeeding difficulties (e.g. inadequate supply) Increased minor depressive symptoms Diastasis recti (separation of the abdominal muscles) Sleep deprivation	Postpartum depression

Table 5.3 Maternal complications common to all twin pregnancies

Stage	Minor risks	Major risks
First trimester	Minor malformation	Miscarriage Structural malformation Aneuploidy
Second and third trimesters	Intrauterine growth restriction	Fetal death in utero, stillbirth
Intrapartum	Non-reassuring cardiotocograph	Twin 2 at increased perinatal risk compared with twin 1
Postpartum	Minor sequelae of prematurity: transient tachypnoea, low blood glucose, hypothermia, delayed oral-feeding ability, lower school performance compared with peers	Major sequelae of prematurity: respiratory distress syndrome; bronchopulmonary dysplasia and oxygen requirement; intraventricular haemorrhage; cerebral palsy; attentional, conduct and behavioural disorders

Table 5.4 Fetal complications common to all twin pregnancies

are ideally cared for in an obstetric unit where the appropriate expertise is available (e.g. a twin's clinic). All twin pregnancies have the same general risks listed below. In addition, monochorionic twins have additional risks due to the shared placenta.

Preterm labour This is the most common risk of twin pregnancy. Half of all twin births are premature due to preterm labour. However, in most cases, the birth is late premature (the average gestational age for twin birth is 35–36 weeks). In 10% of cases, the twins are born extremely premature, at < 28 weeks' gestation.

Twin-to-twin transfusion syndrome This complication is specific to monochorionic pregnancies. It is characterised by unbalanced fetal transfusion between the twins, resulting from unbalanced placental vascular communication in the developing placenta. It characteristically presents in the mid-trimester; therefore, serial US surveillance begins from 16 weeks.

Twin-to-twin transfusion syndrome (TTTS) is classified according to Quintero's stage (**Table 5.5**). These stages determine the management, alongside the wishes of the parents.

Quintero's stage	Findings	Management	Outcomes
1	Donor: oligohydramnios (deepest vertical pocket <2 cm) Recipient: polyhydramnios (deepest vertical pocket >8 cm)	Close observation Laser photocoagulation of placental communications in some centres	86% survival 75% remain stable or regress without intervention
2	Donor: absent bladder Recipient: distended bladder	Laser photocoagulation of placental communications in many centres Amnioreduction in some centres: likely to be required to be serial and outcomes poorer, subsequent laser treatment more difficult	75–80% survival
3	Abnormal Doppler studies	Laser photocoagulation Amnioreduction in centres without expertise in laser treatment	Stages 3–5: 70–100% mortality without intervention
4	Hydrops fetalis	Laser photocoagulation Amnioreduction in centres without expertise in laser treatment	Almost 100% mortality without intervention. Low survival, even with treatment
5	Death (of one or both)	–	50% or 100% mortality Very high rates of major disability in survivors

*The five stages are classified by severity, according to US findings.

Table 5.5 Quintero staging*

Pathogenesis All monochorionic twins have anastomoses (connections between blood vessels of each twin) in their shared placenta. In 15% of cases, these include unbalanced arteriovenous anastomoses, through which one twin (the donor) pumps extra blood to the other twin (the recipient). Consequently, the donor becomes hypovolaemic with an activated renin–aldosterone–angiotensin axis favouring salt and water retention, thereby exacerbating further the hypervolaemia and circulatory overload of the recipient twin.

Management This occurs in specialised tertiary centres. Stage 1 can be observed, but more advanced stages are treated with fetoscopic surgery and ablation of the communicating vessels (amnioreduction, amniocentesis and deliberate removal of excess amniotic fluid, from the polyhydramniotic side is less effective but is performed when fetoscopic ablation is unavailable).

Prognosis Twin-to-twin transfusion syndrome is associated with various adverse fetal outcomes. These range from discordant growth and haemoglobin results to myocardial dysfunction, ventricular hypertrophy, valvular regurgitation and cardiac failure leading to hydrops fetalis and fetal death. Survivors are at increased risk of cerebral palsy and neurological disability resulting from brain injury due to circulatory challenges and spontaneous or iatrogenic prematurity.

Twin anaemia–polycythaemia sequence Like TTTS, twin anaemia polycythaemia sequence is a monochorionic-specific complication caused by unbalanced anastomoses. However, unlike in TTTS, these anastomoses are small, leading to chronic transfusion of red cells into the recipient twin. Twin anaemia polycythaemia sequence is less common than TTTS as a spontaneous event (5%) but occurs after 15% of laser photocoagulation procedures for TTTS.

Chronic transfusion causes polycythaemia (an abnormally high concentration of red blood cells) and hyperviscosity in the recipient and anaemia in the donor. Consequences include those listed for TTTS.

Management Treatment options for twin anaemia polycythaemia sequence are similar to those for TTTS, with the addition of intrauterine transfusion to the donor twin.

Prognosis The odds of survival are superior to those for TTTS, ranging from 75% with observation alone to close to 100% with laser photocoagulation and intrauterine transfusion.

Other monochorionic twin risks Because of their shared placenta, monochorionic twins are at higher risk than dichorionic twins of malformations and fetal death in utero. Aneuploidy is more common in monochorionic twins, as abnormal embryos are more likely to divide abnormally and form monochorionic twins than euploid ones. Other risks are selective intrauterine growth restriction (IUGR; see page 115) and twin anaemia polycythaemia syndrome; specific surveillance is required for these conditions.

5.3 Congenital malformations

Congenital physical anomalies significant enough to be recognised at or soon after birth are termed as congenital malformations (or birth defects). They affect about 4% of newborns. In 1.5% of these cases, the malformation is considered major and results in lifelong disability. Generally, malformations arising early in embryonic or fetal life are major, whereas those arising later in the pregnancy are minor. Minor malformations tend to be of cosmetic rather than functional significance.

Congenital malformations are often a feature of chromosomal abnormalities such as aneuploidy (the presence of an abnormal number of chromosomes in each cell). Chromosomal abnormalities that are incompatible with life usually lead to miscarriage or fetal death in utero. Fetuses affected by other chromosomal abnormalities, most commonly Patau syndrome (trisomy 13) (**Table 5.6**), Edwards syndrome (trisomy 18) (**Table 5.7**) Down syndrome (trisomy 21) (**Table 5.8**), and Turner's syndrome (**Table 5.9**) can survive to birth.

Investigations

If a result from maternal serum screening, or non-invasive prenatal testing is in the high-risk category (which is different

Stage visible	Features
Antenatal biochemistry	↓ pregnancy-associated plasma protein-A ↓ human chorionic gonadotrophin
Antenatal US	Holoprosencephaly (failure of the forebrain to develop into hemispheres) Cyclopia Ventriculomegaly Enlarged cisterna magna Microcephaly Cleft lip and palate Neural tube defect Omphalocele Renal and urogenital malformations Single umbilical artery Polydactyly and flexion deformity of the fingers Early intrauterine growth restriction
Postnatal	Microcephaly (small head circumference) Microphthalmia (small eyes) Cleft lip and palate Sloping forehead Absent eyebrows Low-set, dysplastic ears Prominent occiput Clenched fists and polydactyly 'Rocker bottom' feet Umbilical hernia Undescended or abnormal testes

*The most common malformations are craniofacial, cerebral and genitourinary. Major structural malformations are visible on US antenatally. Characteristic facial appearance and dysmorphism are obvious postnatally.

Table 5.6 Patau syndrome (trisomy 13): features*

for each test), the woman is referred for antenatal counselling before diagnostic investigations are offered (**Figure 5.1**). The routine mid-trimester US scan at 18–22 weeks (the '20-week scan') is offered to all pregnant women for the detection of major (and some minor) malformations.

Ultrasound (US) detection rates for congenital malformation vary according to body system. They are highest for major malformations of the central nervous system such as anencephaly and spina bifida (close to 100%) (**Figures 5.3** and **5.4**),

Stage visible	Features
Antenatal biochemistry	↓ pregnancy-associated plasma protein-A and human chorionic gonadotrophin
Antenatal US	Choroid plexus cysts (significant only if another US marker is present) Congenital talipes equinovarus (club foot) Single umbilical artery Omphalocele Diaphragmatic hernia Renal and cardiac defects Polyhydramnios Early intrauterine growth restriction
Postnatal	Dolichocephaly (longer head relative to width) Low-set ears Micrognathia (undersized jaw) Clenched hand with overriding 4th and 5th digits Short sternum and wide-set nipples Congenital talipes equinovarus (club foot)

*The most common malformations are cardiac and renal. Major structural malformations are visible on US antenatally. Characteristic facial appearance and dysmorphism are obvious postnatally.

Table 5.7 Edwards syndrome (trisomy 18): features*

lower for malformation of the cardiovascular system (about 50%) and lowest for malformations of the musculoskeletal system (roughly 20%).

Hard markers These are malformations seen on US that indicate a high likelihood of a specific chromosomal abnormality. For example, duodenal atresia is a hard marker that appears on US as a double gastric bubble; one-third of fetuses with this feature have Down syndrome. Omphalocele (the presence of abdominal organs in a sac outside the body) is another hard marker. It is associated with a 30% chance of aneuploidy and a 30% chance of another structural malformation.

Soft markers These are malformations seen on US that increase the likelihood of aneuploidy but not enough for the pregnancy to be categorised as being at high risk of this abnormality.

Stage visible	Features
Antenatal biochemistry	↓ pregnancy-associated plasma protein-A ↑ human chorionic gonadotrophin
Antenatal US	Double-bubble sign of duodenal atresia Congenital cardiac defects Thickened nuchal fold (visible as wider area of nuchal translucency) Ventriculomegaly Aberrant right subclavian artery Echogenic bowel Absent nasal bone Short long bones Intracardiac echogenic focus (significant only if another US marker present) Pyelectasis (significant only if another US marker present)
Postnatal	Epicanthic folds Flat midface Low set ears Single palmar crease Umbilical hernia Sandal gap between the big toe and other toes Hypotonia Intestinal stenosis Congenital heart defects (e.g. atrioventricular septal defect) Intellectual disability of varying severity Predisposition to leukaemia, hypothyroidism, epilepsy, early-onset Alzheimer's dementia

*The most common malformations are cardiac and gastrointestinal. Major structural malformations are visible on US antenatally. Characteristic facial appearance and dysmorphism are obvious postnatally.

Table 5.8 Down syndrome (trisomy 21): features*

(The exception is in cases of a screening test result that is close to the cut-off point for the high-risk category).

Management

Malformations are generally not treatable antenatally. Parents have two choices:
- Continue the pregnancy with the prospect of neonatal death, disability or (if available) postnatal treatment or surgery
- Terminate the pregnancy

Congenital malformations

Antenatal	Postnatal
Cystic hygroma	Widely spaced eyes
Hydrops fetalis	Low hairline
Thickened nuchal fold (visible as wider area of nuchal translucency)	Low-set ears
	Webbed neck
Congenital cardiac disease, particularly bicuspid aortic valve and aortic coarctation (may be detected postnatally)	Cubitus valgus (forearm angled away from the body)
	Shield-like chest and widely spaced nipples
Horseshoe kidney	Lymphoedema
	Short stature
	Pigmented naevi
	Infertility
	Amenorrhea

*The most common malformations are cardiac and renal. Major structural malformations are visible on US antenatally. Characteristic facial appearance and dysmorphism are noted postnatally, but may be subtle resulting in detection in older childhood or adolescence.

Table 5.9 Turner's syndrome: features*

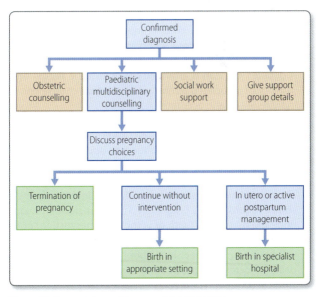

Figure 5.1 Approach to possible congenital malformation.

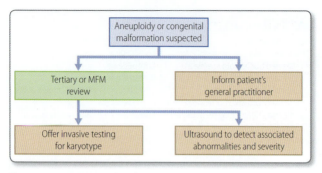

Figure 5.2 Management of confirmed high-risk aneuploidy during pregnancy.

Principles of managing high-risk aneuploidy The general principles of antenatal management of a case of high-risk aneuploidy screening result in addition to standard antenatal care are as follows (**Figure 5.2**):
- After discussion with the woman and her partner about the result and the possible complications of invasive diagnostic testing, chorionic villous sampling (before 14 weeks) or amniocentesis (after 15 weeks) is offered
- A detailed US scan is arranged to confirm the nature and severity of associated abnormalities, so that counselling is individualised and accurate
- Antenatal counselling is provided by a specialist in maternofetal medicine, a neonatologist and other professionals working in paediatric specialities, as appropriate (e.g. a cardiac surgeon if congenital cardiac disease is an associated condition)
- The woman and her partner are supported in their informed choice regarding the pregnancy. They may decide to continue the pregnancy (with or without further testing) or to terminate it. If they wish to continue the pregnancy, they will have to make decisions about plans for extrauterine palliative care (also called comfort care) or resuscitation and surgical correction of defects

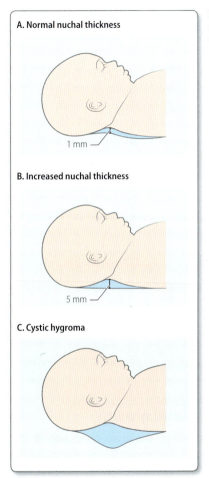

Figure 5.3 Increased nuchal translucency and cystic hygroma.

- If the pregnancy is continued, the woman's plans for monitoring during labour, and her wishes regarding caesarean section if intrapartum complications arise, must be discussed ahead of time. This is because affected fetuses often have IUGR (see page 115) with poor reserves, and tolerate labour poorly

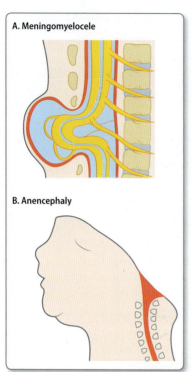

Figure 5.4 Neural tube defects: meningomyelocele and anencephaly.

A. Meningomyelocele

B. Anencephaly

5.4 Disorders of fetal growth

Disorders of fetal growth affect the smallest and largest 10% of fetuses.

The major disorders of fetal growth are excessively large size, excessively small size and divergence from the expected growth trajectory. Fetal growth is of interest as a marker for risk of fetal compromise and poor perinatal outcome.

Investigations

If a disorder of fetal growth is suspected from serial measurements of symphyseal-fundal height (SFH), US scan is used to

Disorders of fetal growth 109

assess the size of the fetus and carry out Doppler studies to detect any abnormalities.

Fetal biometry Ultrasound is used to measure fetal growth. Calipers are placed at predetermined points on the fetal head, to measure head circumference (HC); the abdomen, to measure abdominal circumference (AC); and the femur, to measure

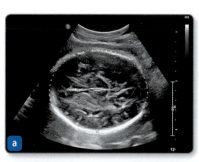
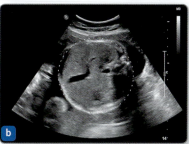
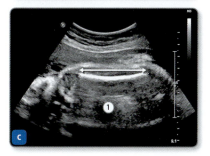

Figure 5.5 Fetal biometry. (a) Head circumference (white dotted line) and BPD. (b) Abdominal circumference (white dotted line. (c) Femur measurement ①.

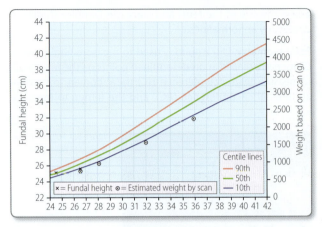

Figure 5.6 Growth chart showing the growth trajectory for a small-for-gestational-age fetus.

> **Clinical insight**
>
> Detection of disorders of fetal growth improves outcomes. For example, in identified cases, IUGR is associated with a four-fold increase in the relative risk of stillbirth, whereas this goes up to an eight-fold increase if the condition is present but undetected and not surveilled.

its length (**Figure 5.5**). The measurements are used to estimate fetal weight, which is plotted on a growth chart (**Figure 5.6**).

The 'symmetry' of the fetus, represented by the ratio of HC to AC, is monitored over time. Values that follow the normal trajectory are generally reassuring. If the fetus is of normal size, this result means that liver growth and accumulation of intra-abdominal fat are normal, indicating healthy placental function. If the fetus is small, symmetrical growth suggests a cause other than a poorly functioning placenta such as constitutional, genetic, infective or other causes.

Asymmetrical growth In cases of asymmetrical growth, the head grows at a normal rate while growth of the rest of the body falls behind. This indicates that the fetus is directing its energy towards development and maintenance of the brain and heart at the expense of growth of the liver and muscle and storage of abdominal fat, which is the fetal response to placental insufficiency (inadequate fetal nutrition via the placenta). Consequently, AC fails to increase in proportion to the increase in HC.

These findings are often accompanied by Doppler results indicating changes in fetal blood flow to compensate for a poorly functioning placenta.

Doppler assessment

Doppler studies are used to assess for abnormalities in the uterine, placental or fetal circulations that cause or indicate a fetal growth disorder (see page 110).

Uterine artery Doppler studies of blood flow through the uterine artery are done to assess whether blood flow to the placenta is of low resistance, as it should be in a healthy pregnancy, or high resistance, which increases the risk of complications including growth restriction and pre-eclampsia. Therefore, uterine artery Doppler studies are required for pregnancies considered at high risk of these complications, due to maternal history or pregnancy-related risk factors. The presence of a 'notch' in the second trimester is associated with poor placentation and reflects high placental resistance due to inadequate villous architecture (**Figure 5.7**). The utility of uterine artery Doppler has not been demonstrated past the second trimester.

Umbilical artery The finding of an increased ratio of

> **Clinical insight**
>
> In pregnancies with IUGR, umbilical artery Doppler studies reduce the risk of perinatal death while reducing unnecessary interventions, thereby allowing deliveries to occur at the optimal time. However, they are less useful for gestations over 34 weeks, because the whole placental bed is larger and may remain normal despite fetal compromise. For this reason if the umbilical artery Doppler study is abnormal after 34 weeks, this is a particularly concerning finding.
>
> Other Dopplers are used in detection and surveillance of fetuses who are IUGR or at risk of IUGR because they increase detection rates. These include the middle cerebral artery Doppler and the cerebroplacental ratio.

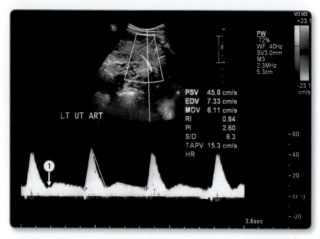

Figure 5.7 Uterine artery Doppler results for a pregnancy of 21 weeks' gestation, showing ① a diastolic 'notch'.

systolic to diastolic flow (SD ratio) on an umbilical artery Doppler study (**Figure 5.8**) reflects high placental bed resistance due to maldeveloped or damaged placental villous architecture. Over time, this progresses to absent end-diastolic flow (**Figure 5.9**) as placental function worsens.

Reversed diastolic flow (**Figure 5.10**) occurs when placental resistance exceeds fetal diastolic blood pressure and blood flows back towards the fetus in diastole. This is severely abnormal and mandates timely delivery by caesarean section.

Middle cerebral artery A decrease in middle cerebral artery resistance demonstrates that the fetus is preferentially streaming blood to its brain. This is a sign of the 'redistribution' of blood to vital organs that occurs when placental resistance is high (**Figure 5.11**).

Ductus venosus An abnormal Doppler result for the ductus venosus reflects fetal decompensation, acidosis and heart

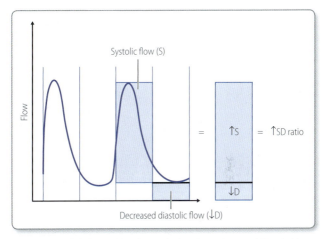

Figure 5.8 Umbilical artery Doppler results showing an increased SD ratio (a) due to a decrease in diastolic flow (b).

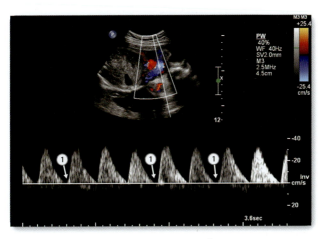

Figure 5.9 Umbilical artery Doppler results showing (1) absent end-diastolic flow.

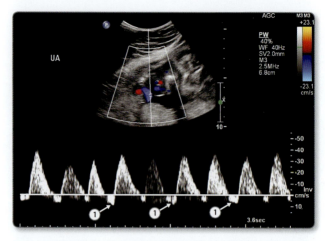

Figure 5.10 Umbilical artery Doppler results showing ① reversed end-diastolic flow.

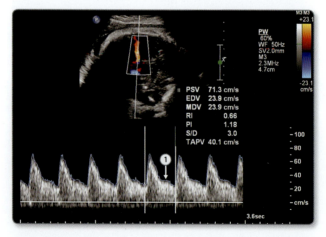

Figure 5.11 Middle cerebral artery Doppler results showing ① low-resistance artery circulation (high diastolic flow) and therefore, signs of redistribution of blood flow.

failure and predicts imminent fetal death. It reflects a reversal of blood flow away from the fetus. Loss or reversal of the 'a' wave (representing atrial contraction) occurs in cases of established acidosis and right heart failure. This is usually accompanied by other abnormalities, such as umbilical venous pulsation, late decelerations on cardiotocography (CTG) and an abnormal biophysical profile (see page 37). If the fetus is viable, delivery is expedited by urgent caesarean section, because this Doppler pattern correlates strongly with perinatal mortality.

Small-for-gestational-age fetus

A small-for-gestational-age (SGA) fetus has an estimated body weight (based on US measurements) below the 10th centile for its gestational age but is otherwise healthy with stable growth trajectory and normal Doppler results. Cases are identified when serial measurements are plotted on a growth chart, as shown in **Figure 5.6**. In the absence of severe small size (less than 3rd centile), aneuploidy or suspicion of infection, the majority of cases are constitutional and concordant with the size of the parents who are also small and the excess in perinatal risk is minimal. Monthly assessments of growth are indicated to ensure the diagnosis has been made correctly and timed birth from 38 weeks is recommended.

Intrauterine growth restriction

This is characterised by the failure of a fetus to meet its genetic potential for growth. It overlaps with SGA to some extent. Most fetuses with IUGR are also SGA (i.e. below the 10th centile in weight for gestational age). However, IUGR also affects fetuses whose growth is within the

> **Clinical insight**
>
> Fetuses that are small, but also smaller than they should be, are often difficult to separate from healthy small-for-gestational-age (SGA) babies with certainty. Therefore, in practice, all cases of SGA are followed. Fetuses that remain within the normal range but have not grown to their potential can be missed and presumed healthy if attention is not paid to other signs including falling growth rate over time, asymmetrical growth (see below) and abnormal Doppler studies. These fetuses require surveillance also.

Fetus	Description	Clinical significance
A	Normal weight but with falling interval growth between serial US scans and small abdominal circumference relative to head circumference	Fetus A has IUGR but is not yet absolutely small/less than 10th centile Falling growth and 'skinny' abdomen (like that of an adult on a weight-loss diet) suggests placental insufficiency and risk of fetal compromise Further history and examination required to determine cause, with monitoring of the pregnancy and timed delivery
B	On 8th centile, with parents of small stature and weight Growth shown on US is stable and abdomen well grown	Fetus B is objectively a small-for-gestational-age fetus but does not have IUGR; it is at minimal or no excess perinatal risk Some fetuses below 10th centile for estimated fetal weight are constitutionally small (i.e. small due to its genetic potential)

Table 5.10 Comparison of two fetuses, A and B

normal range but have failed to reach their genetic potential. The features of both conditions are compared in **Table 5.10**, using two different fetuses as examples.

Aetiology

The causes of IUGR are classified as placental, constitutional, fetal, infective and environmental (**Table 5.11**).

Clinical features

The two major patterns of IUGR are:
- **Symmetrical:** the whole fetus has proportions in concordance
- **Asymmetrical:** the abdomen is small in proportion to the head suggesting that fat deposition has been halted as energy is instead directed towards growth of vital organs such as the brain

Most cases of IUGR are asymmetrical and due to placental insufficiency. However, other causes are considered if the fetus is very small (below the 3rd centile especially), shows growth

Type	Causes	Pattern
Placental (60% of cases)	Deficient placental invasion in first trimester Abnormal location of placenta (e.g. placenta praevia) Abnormal cord (e.g. membranous, two-vessel)	Asymmetrical Associated US findings reflecting placental insufficiency and compensatory change (e.g. abnormal Doppler patterns or oligohydramnios)
Constitutional (25% of cases)	Genetic potential	Symmetrical US findings normal Usually above 5th centile
Fetal (5% of cases)	Chromosomal abnormality Structural malformation	Symmetrical Associated morphological abnormalities
Infective (5% of cases)	TORCH* organisms (toxoplasmosis, cytomegalovirus in particular)	Symmetrical Associated markers of fetal infection
Environmental (5% of cases)	Medication or substance use (prescribed drugs, smoking, alcohol consumption, amphetamine or cocaine misuse) Lifestyle factors (extreme exercise or nutritional deficiency)	Generally asymmetrical

*TORCH, toxoplasmosis, other (varicella-zoster virus, syphilis and parvovirus), rubella, cytomegalovirus and herpes.

Table 5.11 Intrauterine growth restriction: types and causes

in a symmetrical pattern or lacks other signs of placental insufficiency (e.g. abnormal Doppler patterns or oligohydramnios).

Diagnostic approach
The approach to diagnosing IUGR requires the following:
- **History:** the presence of risk factors (**Table 5.12**), maternal reporting of abdominal growth (e.g. compared with other pregnancies) and fetal movement patterns

Category	Factors
Maternal	Extremes of maternal age (<18 or >40 years) Chronic disease Malnutrition, malabsorption History of intrauterine growth restriction in previous pregnancy Drug or alcohol use, smoking
Fetal	Abnormal placentation: bipartite, circumvallate, praevia, marginal cord or membranous cord insertion Abnormal fetus: aneuploidy, genetic disorder, structural malformation
Pregnancy	Hyperemesis Poor gestational weight gain Pre-eclampsia Pregnancy-induced hypertension

Table 5.12 Intrauterine growth restriction: risk factors

- **Examination:** clinical examination to assess fetal size, SFH and liquor volume
- **Investigation:** US examination to measure fetal growth, estimate fetal weight, and assess symmetry, Doppler patterns and amniotic fluid index

Investigations

Intrauterine growth restriction is suspected if any of the following are found on US:
- Falling interval growth between serial scans, dropping centiles over time (especially by 30 or more percentage points)
- Absolute size below the 10th centile (odds ratio 38.1 times of IUGR)
- Abdominal circumference below the 10th centile (odds ratio 18.4 times of IUGR)
- Asymmetry (HC>30 percentile points higher than AC)

Women with risk factors for IUGR require two or three US scans in the third trimester. These are needed to determine whether the fetus is small and to track the trend over time (to detect 'falling growth'). Measurement of SFH (the 'tape measure test') detects only 40–50% of cases of IUGR.

Management

For all cases of IUGR, ongoing surveillance until birth is recommended to reduce the risk of adverse outcomes, such as meconium liquor, caesarean section for non-reassuring CTG in labour, low Apgar score and fetal death in utero (FDIU).

> **Clinical insight**
>
> Fetal growth cannot meaningfully be monitored by US at intervals of <14 days. Over such a short period, any potential growth would be less than the margin of error of the technique. Therefore, the difference between the serial measurements would not necessarily represent growth. Conversely, repeat assessments of growth are no more than 4 weeks apart.

Delivery Regarding birth, the two major considerations are timing and mode. If the pregnancy is at term, timing of delivery is straightforward because delivery is indicated. Before term, the general principle is that the shorter the gestation, the more serious and significant the abnormal findings need to be to justify early delivery and the associated complications of prematurity and low birthweight. Most hospitals have established protocols.

If Doppler results show absent or reversed flow in the umbilical artery or an abnormal ductus venosus pattern, delivery by caesarean section is indicated. If the Doppler results are normal, women may be offered a trial of labour. However, compared with women whose pregnancies are unaffected by IUGR, they are more likely to require caesarean section for non-reassuring fetal status in labour. This is because fetuses with IUGR have lower physiological reserves than normally growing fetuses of the same gestational age.

Macrosomia

Macrosomia is defined by fetal weight greater than the 90th centile for the given gestation. It is more common in pregnancies complicated by maternal obesity, excessive gestational weight gain and diabetes (either pre-existing or gestational). It also occurs without obvious antecedent cause, and much more rarely, due to overgrowth syndromes such as Beckwith-Wiedemann syndrome. Macrosomia increases the risk of shoulder dystocia, perineal trauma and caesarean delivery.

> **Guiding principle**
>
> Although the likelihood of shoulder dystocia increases with birthweight, half of all cases occur when the baby's birthweight is in the normal range. All accoucheurs should practise shoulder dystocia drills regularly.

Macrosomic fetuses carried by women with diabetes are also at increased risk of stillbirth at term.

Management

Once a macrosomic fetus is identified the antecedent cause is determined so that potential complications can be identified. Management is then planned accordingly in the pregnancy (e.g. diabetes care). Large babies who are delivered a week or two before their due date are less likely to be very large at birth as they have had less time to grow and this translates into lower risks of caesarean section and other complications.

Pregnancies unaffected by diabetes In the absence of maternal diabetes or hyperglycaemia, macrosomia makes little change to perinatal risk overall, and unless the estimated birthweight is very large (≥ 5 kg), vaginal delivery is a reasonable option. An experienced accoucheur attends the birth, and the team should be prepared to manage potential shoulder dystocia.

Diabetes in pregnancy It is appropriate to monitor fetal well-being in the latter portion of the third trimester of pregnancies affected by diabetes. However, no high-level evidence is available to guide practice on the optimal timing of initiation, method or frequency of monitoring. Additionally, interpretation is complicated by the diabetes itself; for example, the amniotic fluid index is normal or even increased due to fetal polyuria arising from hyperglycaemia.

The cut-off point for offering caesarean section because of the increased risk of shoulder dystocia is an estimated weight of 4500 g. This is because the diabetic infant has altered anthropometric measurements and is relatively broad-shouldered compared with a baby with an equivalent birthweight. Similar caveats apply as for pregnancies not complicated by diabetes.

The paediatrician must be made aware of the presence of maternal diabetes and the baby's birthweight. The infant is at risk of short-term neonatal hypoglycaemia and neonatal blood glucose levels need to be monitored. In the long term, macrosomia and maternal hyperglycaemia are associated with increased risk of metabolic syndrome in later life.

5.5 Malpresentation

Presentation is defined by the part of the fetus closest to the cervix. Malpresentation is any presentation that is non-cephalic.

Non-cephalic presentation is common before term, and unless the woman enters labour, it is not clinically relevant. At 28 weeks, one in four fetuses are breech. By term, this figure falls to 1 in 20, because most cases resolve without intervention.

Types

Breech is the commonest malpresentation, and may be compatible with vaginal birth (**Figure 5.12**). Other malpresentations include non-longitudinal lies such as transverse, shoulder, arm, funic (involving the umbilical cord) and compound (involving more than one fetal body part). These positions are incompatible with vaginal delivery; caesarean section is required.

Management

Most malpresentations seen before 36 weeks resolve of their own accord (spontaneous version), unless there is another cause. These include an obstructing fibroid, fetal abnormality or placenta praevia (see page 134).

Weeks 23–25 At periviable gestations (weeks 23–25), vaginal delivery of a fetus in a non-longitudinal uterine lie is possible if it is small enough to fold and fit through the dilating cervix, particularly if the membranes are intact and the woman multiparous.

After 36 weeks Near term, any malpresentation is confirmed by US. In the absence of any other contraindication to a vaginal birth, the following options are discussed with the woman.

Fetal and placental complications during pregnancy

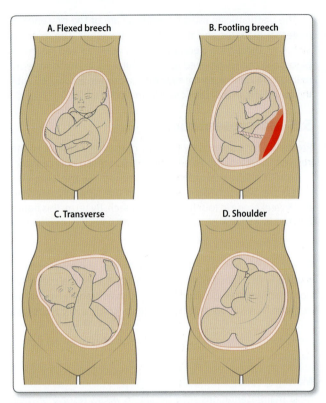

Figure 5.12 Types of malpresentation. Flexed breech presents with a well-applied presenting part to the cervix (the buttocks) which are similar in size to the fetal head. Footling breech has a poorly applied presenting part and has a risk of cord prolapse during labour. Persistent transverse presentations cannot be born vaginally. Shoulder presentations are when the shoulder is the leading presenting part.

External cephalic version This is the safest and most commonly used option for a planned vaginal birth (**Figure 5.13**). Terbutaline aids uterine relaxation, if required. A real-time US scan is used to confirm the change of position in successful procedures. The major risks are:
- Local abdominal pain
- Minor bruising

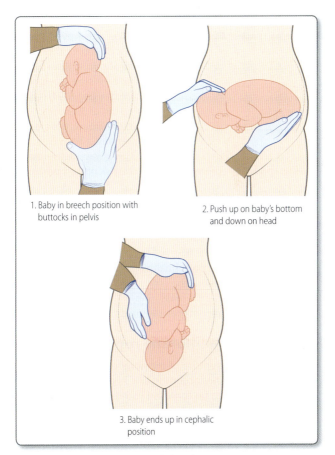

Figure 5.13 External cephalic version for breech presentation.

- Failure (more likely in primigravida or women with obesity, and in cases of anterior placenta, oligohydramnios, extended legs or engaged buttocks)
- A 1-in-200 risk of urgent caesarean for abnormalities on CTG

Other complications, such as placental abruption, are rare.

> **Clinical insight**
>
> It is essential for all obstetric staff to maintain the knowledge and skills needed to manage a birth with the baby still in the breech position. This is because breeches occasionally remain undetected until labour is well advanced.

Caesarean section If the fetus has not moved to the cephalic position, either spontaneously or with external cephalic version, caesarean section (see page 194) can be carried out at 39 weeks.

Unless labour progresses very rapidly, a baby in a footling breech position (see **Figure 5.12**) is always delivered by caesarean section. This is because of the risk of cord prolapse.

Planned vaginal breech birth This is offered if the obstetrician and other members of the team are experienced in the procedure and if the following factors apply:
- The woman is multiparous
- The fetus is of normal size
- The pregnancy has been healthy
- Labour is spontaneous
- The cardiotocograph is reassuring

If these conditions are not met, caesarean section is indicated.

5.6 Preterm membrane rupture

Preterm prelabour rupture of membranes (PPROM) is a rupture of the membranes occurring at < 37 completed weeks of gestation. It is not to be confused with prelabour rupture of membranes (PROM), which is experienced by 15% of women at term. The main risks of PPROM are maternal and fetal infection (chorioamnionitis) and spontaneous labour and the sequelae of prematurity. Overall, 80% of women with PPROM give birth within 7 days of the diagnosis.

> **Guiding principle**
>
> Generally, unless infection is present, the further the pregnancy is from term, the less likely spontaneous labour is to occur after PPROM. However, if labour intervenes, infection should be strongly suspected.

Chorioamnionitis refers to overt infection in the amniotic fluid around the fetus; it is a severe infection associated with maternal and fetal sepsis and is only relieved by birth.

Aetiology

Precipitating factors for PPROM include uterine overdistension, cervical shortening, and factors that cause membrane inflammation and rupture, e.g. infection (commonly subclinical) and recurrent antepartum haemorrhage. Infections such as bacterial vaginosis and the major sexually transmitted infections are associated with PPROM.

Clinical features

Signs of PPROM include:
- A 'washed out' vagina on speculum examination (normal leukorrhoea has been washed away by the passage of amniotic fluid)
- Fresh liquor pooling in the posterior fornix on speculum examination
- Liquor emerging from the external cervical os when the woman coughs on speculum examination
- A positive result from a rupture of membranes test

Tachycardia is a sign of fetal infection.

Diagnostic approach

Preterm prelabour rupture of membranes is suspected if there is a history of fluid leakage. This can be subtle if the membrane defect is small and high (a hind-water leak).

The woman is examined to assess uterine tenderness (indicating infection) and contractions (indicating labour). Fetal presentation and lie are determined. A sterile speculum is used to carry out a vaginal examination to confirm PPROM, assess the colour and odour of the liquor for signs of infection (purulent or offensive liquor indicates chorioamnionitis), determine cervical dilation and exclude cord prolapse.

Investigations

A full blood examination and C-reactive protein (CRP) test are required. Increases in neutrophil count and CRP concentration suggest infection. A urine specimen and a

> **Clinical insight**
>
> Unless delivering the baby, never carry out a digital cervical examination in cases of PPROM. Digital cervical examination increases the risk of infection.

high vaginal swab are sent for culture to screen for pathogenic organisms (most notably group B *Streptococcus*). A formal US scan to assess fetal growth, presentation and the amount of remaining liquor provides further information needed to formulate the management plan for delivery and neonatal care.

Management

The aims of management are to gain gestational maturity, if this is safe, and to minimise the risk of infection and associated complications. The woman is admitted to hospital; this would be a tertiary centre if gestation is < 32–34 weeks. Drugs used to manage PPROM are antibiotics, betamethasone (to improve neonatal outcomes) and nifedipine (sometimes used to suppress labour) (**Table 5.13**). Maternal temperature and liquor colour are checked four times daily. For gestations of over 26–28 weeks, the condition of the fetus is monitored once daily with CTG for 3 days and then twice weekly. For gestations < 28 weeks, fetal condition is assessed by means of the biophysical profile for the first 3 days and then at least twice weekly because the CTG is difficult to interpret at very preterm gestations.

Medication	Dosage	Indication
Erythromycin	250 mg orally four times daily for 10 days	Infection risk, prophylaxis
Ampicillin	2 g IV four times daily for 48 hours, followed by oral amoxicillin	In addition to erythromycin at less than 32 weeks, infection risk
Betamethasone	11.4 mg intramuscularly, repeated in 24 hours	At <34 weeks to reduce respiratory distress and complications of prematurity
Nifedipine (only after discussion with senior colleague)	20 mg in three doses 30 minutes apart, followed by 20 mg three times daily	Facilitates in utero transfer

Table 5.13 Preterm prelabour rupture of membranes: medications used in management

The woman is advised to notify to the hospital if she notices any symptoms of infection, such as abdominal pain, fever, flu-like symptoms or a change in liquor (to offensive or green), or if she has any contractions or concerns about the well-being of the baby (e.g. arising from reduced fetal movements). Fetal growth is monitored with serial US scans, because SFH is inaccurate in cases of ruptured membranes.

Delivery This is indicated when the risk of chorioamnionitis (see page 154) outweighs the risk of prematurity. Chorioamnionitis develops at any point, but is most common soon after the rupture of membranes and, for this reason, initial observation is in hospital. Delivery is indicated at or past 37 weeks and delivery mode is based on usual obstetric indications.

5.7 Preterm labour

Preterm labour is labour before 37 weeks' gestation. Many insults, including retroplacental bleeding, infection, PPROM, uterine overdistension and maternal illness, can activate the labour cascade. Often, the cause is unclear.

Threatened preterm labour (contractions before 37 weeks without dilation of the cervix) is a common cause of antenatal review. Most women with threatened preterm labour (contractions before term) do not go on to give preterm birth.

Diagnostic approach

The diagnosis of preterm labour requires the presence of uterine contractions and progressive cervical change. Therefore, it is a diagnosis in retrospect, taking up valuable time that could be used for the treatment and transfer of women in true preterm labour. For this reason, clinical triage and predictive testing is used to streamline care to those most likely to benefit.

> **Guiding principle**
>
> Gestation is a surrogate indicator for the obstetric goal of delivering a baby in the best possible condition in the most appropriate setting at the optimal time. They may mean that, after appropriate transfer and maternal treatment, delivery rather than continued pregnancy is the safest option for the fetus.

Fetal fibronectin This test is used to rule out preterm labour. Fetal fibronectin is a protein that adheres the amniotic sac to the uterine lining. Therefore, its presence in secretions obtained by cervical swab indicates disturbance of this connection and increased risk of preterm birth.

A woman with symptoms of preterm labour (i.e. regular contractions) and a negative fetal fibronectin test result has a >95% chance that birth will not occur in the following fortnight. However, a positive result does not mean that labour will occur.

Investigations

Screening for possible precipitating infections requires full blood examination, urine culture and vaginal swab (to obtain specimen of discharge for microscopy and culture). If available, a US scan is also carried out, because the finding of a long cervix (>3 cm) means that the woman is unlikely to go on to give birth in the next few weeks.

If placental abruption is suspected as a cause for preterm contractions due to vaginal bleeding, Kleihauer–Betke test (a test to measure fetal haemoglobin in the maternal circulation, also called the acid elution test) and a US to assess for retroplacental haematoma are useful because they support clinical suspicion. However, neither is sensitive enough to exclude this diagnosis.

> **Clinical insight**
>
> Although 'inborn' preterm babies (those born in a tertiary centre) have better outcomes than 'outborn' ones (those born outside a tertiary centre), the most dangerous scenario is an unexpected in-transit delivery. Before it is decided to transfer a woman in preterm labour to another centre, it is critical to consider the parity of the woman, the risk of complications associated with birth at the specific gestation, the rate of progress of the labour and the estimated transfer time. In cases of doubt, it is safer that the neonatal team come to the woman rather than she be taken to them.

Management

Management of preterm labour depends on gestation and setting of care (tertiary versus secondary).

After 34 weeks If spontaneous labour occurs after 34 weeks, it is allowed to progress because neonatal outcomes are not improved by delay.

Before 34 weeks Unless there is evidence of abruption (e.g. painful vaginal bleeding), infection or fetal compromise, women in preterm labour are given tocolytic medication to temporarily suppress contractions (**Table 5.14**). This provides additional time for transfer to a specialist unit and administration of betamethasone (two doses 24 hours apart) to accelerate maturation of fetal organs. When the cervix is over 3 cm dilated, tocolysis is likely to fail and labour progresses regardless.

Steroid administration Women in preterm labour are given two doses of steroid (betamethasone; see **Table 5.14**) 24 hours apart to induce production of surfactant in the fetal lungs,

Use	Medications	Adverse effects
Tocolysis	Nifedipine tablets	Hypotension Headache
	Terbutaline	Tachycardia Rarely pulmonary oedema, arrhythmia Avoid IV administration (increased risk of severe side effects) Tachyphylaxis (reduction in response to medication and need for escalating doses) with infusion, so not recommended
Group B *Streptococcus* prophylaxis	Benzylpenicillin	Anaphylaxis (1 in 10,000 to 1 in 100,000 cases)
Prevention of neonatal respiratory distress syndrome	Betamethasone	Hyperglycaemia (clinically significant in women with diabetes) Sleep disturbance Local injection site pain Neurological effects in fetus
Fetal neuroprotection	Magnesium sulphate	Flushing, blurred vision, weakness Hypotension Rarely respiratory arrest

Table 5.14 Preterm labour: medications used in management

thereby reducing the risk of neonatal mortality and morbidity due to respiratory distress syndrome. It also decreases intraventricular haemorrhage, necrotising enterocolitis and other major sequelae of preterm birth through its beneficial effects on respiratory function and cardiovascular stability at birth.

Delivery Women in preterm labour are given IV benzylpenicillin to reduce the risk of early-onset group B streptococcal infection in the neonate. If the gestation is under 30 weeks, magnesium sulphate (see page 147) is given by infusion using the same doses as for eclampsia to reduce the risk of cerebral palsy in the baby.

If the fetal presentation is cephalic, vaginal birth is preferred. If the baby is breech, delivery is usually by caesarean section, because of the risk of entrapment of the head (the largest part of a preterm fetus). However, caesarean may not be possible if labour progresses very rapidly.

Prognosis

Babies born at < 23 weeks survive only very rarely. The likelihood of survival increases with gestational age (**Figure 5.14**).

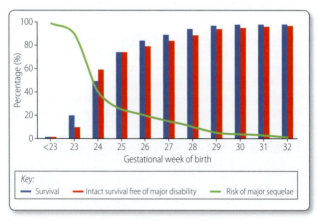

Figure 5.14 Survival and risk of complications in infants born before term.

Major complications are uncommon in babies born in the late preterm period. However, up to a third of these children have subtle identified behavioural or scholastic difficulties at the age of 7 years.

Major complications of preterm birth are:
- Cerebral palsy
- Cognitive impairment
- Seizures
- Chronic lung disease
- Visual and hearing impairment

Minor complications include those arising from neurodevelopmental impairment:
- Attentional difficulties (necessitating additional educational support at school)
- Behavioural problems (e.g. conduct disorder)
- Lower educational attainment in comparison with full-term peers

5.8 Antepartum haemorrhage

Antepartum haemorrhage is bleeding from the genital tract after 20 weeks' gestation. It occurs in 2–5% of all pregnancies, but most instances are minor, i.e. the bleeding is small in amount, and the pregnancy progresses healthily.

If there is uterine scarring (most commonly from a previous caesarean section but sometimes an open myomectomy), the differential diagnosis includes morbidly adherent placenta, because the scar is a site of weakness that the placenta can invade. This is termed placenta accreta, increta or percreta, depending on how much of the scar and uterine wall has been invaded (**Figure 5.15**).

Aetiology

Antepartum haemorrhage is described as 'incidental' or 'accidental'.
- In cases of incidental haemorrhage, the cause of the bleeding is unrelated to the pregnancy (**Table 5.15**)

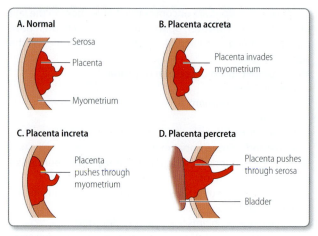

Figure 5.15 Types of morbidly adherent placenta.

Cause	Symptoms	Signs
Vaginal candidiasis	Pruritus, creamy white discharge, pain and burning	Curd-like white discharge, erythematous base below
Cervical ectopy	Painless bleeding, particularly after coitus	Ectopy on speculum examination
Cervical polyp	Painless bleeding, particularly after coitus. Sensation of lump (if very large)	Visible polyp on speculum examination
Cervical dysplasia or malignancy	Bleeding, particularly after coitus. Leg pain, oedema and flank pain in advanced disease	Exophytic mass on speculum examination, abnormal appearance at colposcopy, barrel-shaped cervix in glandular lesions, contact bleeding that may be profuse due to neovascularisation
Urinary or rectal source	Haematuria, bleeding with bowel motions, presence of urinary infection, constipation or haemorrhoids	No blood in vagina. Haematuria. Haemorrhoids. Blood on glove after rectal examination

Table 5.15 Antepartum haemorrhage: incidental causes

Cause	Symptoms	Signs
Marginal bleed	Painful or painless bleeding	Irritable uterine contractions Generally normal cardiotocograph Non-tender uterus
Placental abruption	Painful bleeding with contractions Symptoms of predisposing cause (e.g. pre-eclampsia, trauma)	Irritable uterine contractions, tense uterus Tender uterus, especially over placental site Cardiotocograph ranging from normal to abnormal to pathological Signs of shock Signs of coagulopathy

Table 5.16 Antepartum haemorrhage: accidental causes

Cause	Symptoms	Signs
Placenta praevia	Painless bleeding, spontaneous or provoked by coitus or contractions	Non-tender uterus Bleeding can be profuse Cardiotocograph generally reasonably normal unless massive bleeding or maternal shock Signs of shock
Vasa praevia	Painless bleeding History of low-lying placenta, succenturiate lobe or known vasa praevia Almost always associated with labour or rupture of membranes	Markedly abnormal cardiotocograph out of keeping with relatively minor degree of blood loss

Table 5.17 Antepartum haemorrhage: praevia causes

- In accidental haemorrhage, the bleeding is related to the pregnancy (**Table 5.16**)

Generally, bleeding from placenta praevia is painless (**Table 5.17**), whereas bleeding due to marginal separation or abruption is associated with pain and irritable contractions.

> **Clinical insight**
>
> Placenta accreta is always suspected in the presence of a uterine scar and placenta praevia. A high-quality US study (and occasionally an MRI study) is required to refute or establish the diagnosis with certainty. Missed antenatal diagnosis of placenta accreta substantially increases surgical morbidity and the risk of massive transfusion and unplanned hysterectomy without specialist surgical support.

> **Clinical insight**
>
> Digital vaginal examination is never carried out if there is any doubt about the presence of placenta praevia, because it can provoke profuse haemorrhage.

> **Clinical insight**
>
> In cases of suspected antepartum haemorrhage, sponge forceps and sterile gauze are used during speculum examination to remove blood and clots from the vagina. This enables clear visualisation of the cervix.

Diagnostic approach

The diagnostic approach aims to determine the severity, site, cause and maternal and fetal compromise from the bleeding.

History Enquiries are made about the following.
- Amount of bleeding and whether it is painful or painless
- Number of pads soaked
- Symptoms of ruptured membranes, such as prior clear fluid loss
- Contractions
- Symptoms of shock
- Any known causes (e.g. placenta praevia)

If the bleeding is heavy and conservative management unlikely, a quick '**AMPLE**' (**A**llergies, **M**edicines, **P**ast history, **L**ast oral intake, **E**xercise tolerance) history is taken in preparation for urgent caesarean section.

Examination The DRABC (Danger, Response, Airway, Breathing and Circulation) approach is used. The vital signs are confirmed to be normal. Fluid resuscitation is given if signs of shock are present (in healthy adults, tachycardia is the only sign of shock until late in the process).

Then:
- Abdominal examination is carried out to assess uterine tenderness and contractions

- A speculum examination is done to assess cervical dilation and ongoing bleeding
- Intravenous access is obtained (with simultaneous assessment of whether bleeding is ongoing)
- Cardiotocography is arranged if the pregnancy is over 28 weeks' gestation

Speculum examination Old blood seen on speculum examination is brown or dark, whereas fresh blood is red and trickles from the external cervical os. Occasionally, clot lysis produces a serosanguineous discharge that is mistakenly attributed to rupture of membranes. However, ruptured membranes are unlikely if there is no ongoing fluid leakage and the amniotic fluid index is stable. Small amounts of blood mixed with mucus are termed as a 'show'; this is common at term and is not antepartum haemorrhage.

Investigations

Investigations are carried out to identify the cause of the bleeding, assess for complications and ensure that mother and fetus are well (**Table 5.18**). In all but the most minor of bleeds, at least one 16- to 18-g IV cannula is inserted and blood specimens obtained for full blood examination and group and antibody screen.

Management

Most bleeds are not heavy, and although the cause is frequently not identified, the mother and fetus remain healthy and routine obstetric care is continued. At preterm gestations, management is usually expectant if mother and fetus are well; most affected women are discharged from hospital after 24 hours have passed without a bleed.

Clinical insight

In severe haemorrhage with ongoing blood loss, the consultant obstetrician, operating theatre staff and anaesthetist must be urgently informed. In addition, the local massive transfusion protocol must be activated to facilitate timely access to blood and haematological support.

Investigation	Uses
Full blood examination	Current haemoglobin and platelet counts
Blood group and screen	Excludes irregular red-cell antibodies Allows faster cross-matching or provision of group-specific blood, if required
Coagulation profile	Baseline coagulation status Excludes disseminated intravascular coagulation from profuse haemorrhage and consumptive coagulopathy or pre-existing coagulopathy Low fibrinogen (< 2.5 g/L): requires early replacement with cryoprecipitate, which needs time to thaw
Venous blood gas	Rapid assessment of haematological variables in acute emergencies
US	Placental localisation Exclusion of placenta praevia and vasa praevia Assessment of fetal growth Do not delay delivery for US if the haemorrhage is massive and causing haemodynamic instability

Table 5.18 Antepartum haemorrhage: investigations

At gestations of < 34 weeks, steroid injections of betamethasone are administered to minimise the severity of the potential sequelae of prematurity, in case delivery is indicated by a deteriorating clinical situation. In secondary settings, women with a pregnancy of < 32–34 weeks' gestation are transferred to a tertiary centre with facilities for the care of preterm neonates.

Antenatal care Women who recover from a bleeding episode require optimisation of their depleted iron stores (and thereby haemoglobin levels) with supplementation. If bleeding recurs, fetal growth is monitored with at least monthly US scans to check for IUGR (an associated risk).

Delivery If antepartum haemorrhage occurs at over 37 weeks' gestation, the woman is kept in hospital until birth can be arranged. If fetal status is non-reassuring and the fetus is viable, delivery is carried out quickly by caesarean section. Placenta praevia is always delivered by caesarean section because the placenta obstructs the cervix. This is performed electively any time after 36 weeks, however, if there is severe bleeding, the baby is delivered immediately.

Maternal complications during pregnancy

chapter 6

The health of expectant mothers can be affected by problems that are a consequence of pregnancy, such as antepartum haemorrhage, or an exacerbation by pregnancy of a pre-existing disorder. This pre-existing disorder may be known, such as a woman with chronic hypertension who develops pre-eclampsia in pregnancy; or unknown, such as a woman with gestational diabetes who later develops clinically apparent type 2 diabetes mellitus (T2DM).

The risk of maternal complications is increased by pre-existing chronic disorders, so screening for these disorders and appropriate management is essential.

Clinical insight

Pregnancy is unique because there are two interdependent patients. Complications may put their interests in direct conflict, as the fetus and placenta often contribute to the pathogenesis of maternal complications in pregnancy. For this reason, delivery of the fetus is often the most effective treatment for maternal complications, such as in pre-eclampsia. Generally, the mother's health is prioritised; fetal benefit should not be pursued at the cost of maternal harm.

6.1 Clinical scenario

Liver disease in pregnancy

Presentation

A 38-year-old primigravida with a pregnancy of 39 weeks' gestation presents to the emergency department with nausea, vomiting and upper abdominal pain. She has been feeling unwell with malaise and nausea for 2 days. The history is negative for diarrhoea, sick contacts, autoimmune disease, biliary tract disease, exposure to viral hepatitis, and use of hepatotoxic medication. The course of the pregnancy has been unremarkable to date. Fetal movements have reduced over the past 24 hours.

Examination reveals a confused and unwell woman with yellowish pigmentation of the eyes. Blood pressure (BP) is increased, at 150/90 mmHg. There is no hyper-reflexia (overactive reflexes), clonus (involuntary muscular contractions and relaxations) or generalised oedema. No scratch marks or stigmata of chronic liver disease are present. Apart from upper abdominal tenderness, abdominal examination is unremarkable.

A fetal heart is heard. However, cardiotocography (CTG) shows a non-reactive pattern of activity, and spontaneous decelerations occur with uterine tightenings.

Diagnostic approach

This woman is clinically unwell, jaundiced (as indicated by the scleral icterus) and has an altered mental state. Taken together, these point to a liver disorder serious enough to cause encephalopathy.

Liver disease in pregnancy is broadly divided into cases with a pregnancy-related cause and cases unrelated to pregnancy (**Table 6.1**). Prompt delivery is required to cure the mother in most types of pregnancy-specific liver disease, such as acute fatty liver of pregnancy (AFLP) and pre-eclampsia, whereas delivery is not usually required in cases of liver disease unrelated to pregnancy, as it would not alter the underlying pathology.

In this case, AFLP is more likely than pre-eclampsia because BP is only modestly increased and there are no other signs of pre-eclampsia (hyper-reflexia, clonus and generalised oedema). Non-pregnancy-related causes of liver disease (**Table 6.1**) are clinically unlikely given there is no pre-pregnancy abnormal liver function, intravenous drug use or hepatotoxin consumption.

Acute fetal compromise and poor maternal condition necessitate urgent treatment. Simultaneous assessment, stabilisation and management are required so that delivery can be safely expedited. AFLP is associated with derangements in coagulation and haemostasis. The potential for surgical bleeding mandates rapid assessment and optimisation of the mother's condition, because urgent caesarean section is needed; it is potentially life-saving for mother and baby.

Pregnancy-related causes	Causes unrelated to pregnancy
Pre-eclampsia HELLP syndrome Acute fatty liver of pregnancy Obstetric cholestasis	Autoimmune hepatitis Viral hepatitis (hepatitis A, B or C, Epstein–Barr virus, cytomegalovirus, other) Use of hepatotoxic drugs or other substances Biliary disease Vascular causes (Budd-Chiari syndrome, heart failure)

HELLP, Haemolysis, elevated liver enzymes and low platelets; AFLP, Acute fatty liver of pregnancy.

Table 6.1 Liver disease in pregnancy: causes

Investigations

The woman is cared for in a resuscitation cubicle. Continuous CTG is maintained. Two large-bore IV lines (minimum 16-gauge) are inserted to obtain blood for urgent venous blood gas analysis (which will rapidly provide clinical information), full blood examination, electrolyte and liver function tests, coagulation profile, blood cross-matching, and measurement of glucose, ammonia and inflammatory markers. Because the available history is limited, additional tubes are taken for viral serology, autoantibody testing, paracetamol (acetaminophen) level and bile salts.

An indwelling catheter is inserted. Urinalysis results are 2+ for protein and bilirubin. Finger prick test results show that blood glucose concentration is low, at 1.5 mmol/L.

Preliminary results are obtained from the blood gas analysis and are consistent with rapid laboratory testing, showing mild anaemia [haemoglobin (Hb), 98 g/L], significant thrombocytopaenia (platelet count, 45×10^9/L), elevated liver enzymes (alanine aminotransferase, 446 U/L; aspartate aminotransferase, 256 U/L), increased bilirubin (60 µmol/L), acute kidney injury (creatinine, 120 µmol/L; urea, 18 mmol/L) and autoanticoagulation with evidence of consumption of clotting factors (fibrinogen low, at 1.3 g/L; international normalised ratio prolonged, at 2.3). Spot urine test results show significant proteinuria, with a protein to creatinine ratio of 0.04.

The severity of the woman's condition and the presence of a live fetus with pathological cardiotocographic results warrant urgent delivery by caesarean section. No further fetal investigations are carried out, because this would delay the procedure and the results would not change management.

Management

Consent for caesarean section is obtained from the woman's next of kin, who has accompanied her to hospital because she is too unwell to consent for surgery.

The anaesthetist, intensivist and paediatrician are informed of the case, and plans are made for the woman's urgent transfer to operation theatre. Intravenous glucose is given to correct the hypoglycaemia. The coagulopathy is urgently treated with vitamin K, fresh frozen plasma, platelets and cryoprecipitate.

Caesarean section under general anaesthesia is carried out. A hypotonic neonate in poor condition is delivered and quickly transferred to the neonatal intensive care unit. Surgical haemostasis is achieved. Postoperatively, the woman is admitted to the intensive care unit for ongoing management.

> **Clinical insight**
>
> Acute fatty liver of pregnancy (AFLP) is an obstetric emergency that presents similarly to pre-eclampsia and HELLP syndrome. However, unlike women with these conditions, a woman with AFLP usually looks very unwell, in a way that is out of proportion to the symptoms.

6.2 Hypertension and pre-eclampsia

Hypertension is common in pregnant women. The condition may have been present before pregnancy, as chronic hypertension, or developed during it, as pre-eclampsia or gestational hypertension.

The two pregnancy-related hypertensive disorders are differentiated mainly by the presence or absence of proteinuria (**Figure 6.1**). In a case of new-onset hypertension in pregnancy, gestational hypertension is diagnosed if urinary protein is absent and there is no other evidence of pre-eclampsia. Gestational hypertension is not a benign diagnosis; affected

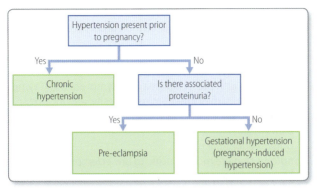

Figure 6.1 Distinguishing chronic hypertension, gestational hypertension and pre-eclampsia during pregnancy.

women remain at risk of developing pre-eclampsia, such as abnormal biochemistry or fetal growth restriction as discussed on page 115. Management is similar for the two disorders.

Pre-eclampsia is defined as new-onset elevated blood pressure persistently >140/90 mmHg, plus any one of the following markers and signs of end-organ dysfunction.

- Proteinuria of greater than a spot protein creatinine ratio of 30 mg/dL or >300 mg in a 24-hour collection in the absence of contamination from leucorrhoea or urinary tract infection
- Haematological abnormalities (e.g. thrombocytopaenia, or haemolysis with anaemia)
- Liver dysfunction (indicated by abnormal liver function test results)
- Neurological abnormalities (e.g. severe headache; photopsia; scotomata; or jitteriness or imminent seizure due to a combination of loss of cerebral autoregulation, hypertensive encephalopathy, lowering of seizure threshold and cerebral oedema)
- Renal impairment (creatinine >90 μmol/L or oliguria)
- Placental dysfunction, indicated by intrauterine growth restriction, placental abruption or abnormal Doppler patterns (see page 111)

By definition, pre-eclampsia can only be diagnosed after 20 weeks' gestation. The rare exception occurs in undiagnosed molar pregnancies.

Clinical features

Many women with pre-eclampsia are asymptomatic. If symptoms are present, they are often non-specific and include:
- Headache
- Blurry vision
- Upper abdominal pain

Symptoms that are more specific to pre-eclampsia are:
- Scotomata
- Rapidly progressive oedema involving the hands or face
- Right upper quadrant pain from hepatic capsular distension
- Jitteriness reflecting neurological irritability and impending seizure

Examination findings are usually normal apart from hypertension with or without pitting oedema of the limbs. Other features of pre-eclampsia include hyper-reflexia (although brisk reflexes are common in normal pregnancy), sustained (three or more) beats of clonus and a tender liver margin. Malignant (severe) hypertension (BP >180/100 mmHg) exceeds cerebral autoregulation and causes cortical blindness from cerebral oedema, as well as eclamptic convulsions and intracranial haemorrhage.

> **Guiding principle**
>
> The HELLP syndrome is a rare form of severe pre-eclampsia characterised by haemolysis, elevated liver enzymes and low platelets. It affects 15% of women with pre-eclampsia. Prompt delivery is curative. Without appropriate treatment, including delivery, women with HELLP syndrome die due to liver rupture and cerebral haemorrhage.

Severe pre-eclampsia This is a progressive disorder and potentially fatal for the mother. The most serious features are:
- Papilloedema, retinal detachment or cortical blindness
- Liver failure or rupture
- Placental abruption or stillbirth
- Seizures, cerebral haemorrhage or cerebral oedema
- Pulmonary oedema

- Renal failure, with or without proteinuria or peripheral oedema
- Disseminated intravascular coagulation

Investigations

Investigations for pre-eclampsia are:
- A full blood examination to detect anaemia resulting from haemolysis and thrombocytopaenia
- Liver function tests (elevated levels of transaminases indicate liver dysfunction)
- Creatinine, urea and electrolyte measurement to detect associated renal impairment (elevated creatinine)
- Uric acid test (concentration increased beyond the gestation-specific reference range in cases of early renal dysfunction)
- Urine for spot quantification of proteinuria

An abnormal cardiotocograph indicates fetal compromise either due to placental dysfunction or the pre-eclamptic illness. The condition of the fetus must be monitored alongside that of the mother.

Management

Management of pre-eclampsia depends on the severity of the disorder, the length of gestation and the condition of mother and fetus. At term (over 37 weeks' gestation), delivery is indicated; before term, the fetus benefits from expectant management. The most common contraindications to expectant management are uncontrolled BP despite maximal antihypertensive medication, deteriorating biochemistry, HELLP syndrome, eclampsia and fetal compromise. There is no reliable way to determine the length of the latent period before the serious complications of pre-eclampsia, including HELLP syndrome and eclampsia, arise. Therefore, close monitoring of maternal and fetal condition is required in all cases.

> **Clinical insight**
>
> If a dipstick urinalysis test is positive for proteinuria, the specimen is sent for formal quantification of proteinuria. This is because the diagnosis of pre-eclampsia cannot be made on the results of dipstick urinalysis alone. A carefully collected midstream urine specimen is sent for testing at the same time, to exclude infection as a cause of mild proteinuria.

Medication	Mode of action	Adverse effects	Onset
Methyldopa	α2-adrenergic receptor agonist and centrally acting antihypertensive Decreases sympathetic outflow	Sedation, depression, parkinsonism, postural hypotension	Very slow
Labetalol	Mixed alpha- and beta-blocker Decreases peripheral vascular resistance and heart rate	Bradycardia, fatigue, scalp tingling, cold extremities, rebound hypertension, sleep disturbance, exacerbation of asthma	Intermediate
Nifedipine	Calcium channel blocker Reduces peripheral vascular tone	Peripheral oedema, headache, postural hypotension, flushing	Immediate release: rapid, especially if chewed Chewing the sustained-release formulation also results in rapid absorption

Table 6.2 Antihypertensive medications used during pregnancy

Hypertension This is treated with a pregnancy-compatible agent (**Table 6.2**). The target BP is about 140/90 mmHg.

Hypertensive urgency This term describes an acute and life-threatening clinical situation in which severe hypertension (>170/110 mmHg) requires management in a high-dependency setting according to the 'stabilise then deliver' principle. The hypertension is controlled with IV antihypertensive drugs

Drug	Administration	Adverse effects	Onset
Labetalol	20 mg/4 mL slow IV push Repeated every 10 minutes until control or five doses (start infusion)	As in Table 6.2 plus hypotension, bradycardia, arrhythmia, non-reassuring cardiotocograph	Rapid
Hydralazine	5–10 mg slow IV push Repeated every 10–20 minutes until control or four doses (start infusion)	Headache, tachycardia, palpitations, flushing, hypotension, non-reassuring cardiotocograph	Rapid

*Oral nifedipine is used if there is no IV access (an oral agent can also be given at the same time as IV treatment for sustained control of hypertension).

Table 6.3 Intravenous antihypertensive medications for acute hypertension in pregnancy*

(**Table 6.3**) to minimise the risk of eclampsia, stroke, intracerebral haemorrhage and placental abruption. If the BP cannot be adequately controlled, the baby is delivered by the safest method for mother and baby. This is not always a caesarean. Magnesium sulphate infusion reduces the risk of an eclamptic seizure (4 g IV loading dose over 20 minutes, followed by 1 g/h infusion), but it is not used instead of antihypertensives because hypertension control is the most important factor in reducing seizure risk.

> **Clinical insight**
>
> The maternal BP must always be reduced gradually. A sharp, precipitous drop is associated with adverse outcomes, such as fetal bradycardia from reduced placental perfusion and maternal collapse.

6.3 Eclampsia

Eclampsia is the generalised seizure activity that occurs in about 1% of women with pre-eclampsia. Uncommonly, it is the presenting feature. Most seizures are brief, and most women have an eclamptic seizure only once.

Investigations

The key investigations are:
- Blood tests (full blood examination, liver function tests, electrolytes, uric acid and coagulation profile)
- Dipstick urinalysis (for rapid assessment of protein levels) and formal quantification of proteinuria by laboratory spot ratio
- Venous blood gas for immediate haemoglobin, electrolytes and glucose; these results rapidly exclude differential diagnoses such as metabolic causes and hypoglycaemia before formal blood tests return from the laboratory

> **Guiding principle**
>
> Differential diagnoses for eclamptic seizure include epilepsy, stroke, cerebral mass lesions and metabolic derangements (e.g. hypoglycaemia). If a woman has recurrent seizures or fails to return to consciousness after a seizure, or if focal neurological symptoms are present, an urgent CT scan of the head is required.

Management

As in cases of severe hypertension, the principle of 'stabilise then deliver' applies. The 'DRABC' approach is followed ensuring that the woman is not left alone while experienced help is summoned, she is in the left lateral position with the cot sides up (and ideally padded to minimise the risk of injury), and her airway is patent. Investigations for eclampsia are carried out; while the hypertension is treated and magnesium sulphate infusion is started for prophylaxis against further seizures (see **Tables 6.2** and **6.3**).

DRABC approach The DRABC approach is a useful mnemonic for all medical emergencies. It stands for:
1. Assess for Danger to yourself and the patient
2. Assess Response
3. Then Airway, Breathing and Circulation

The follow-on letters 'DEFG' represent Don't Ever Forget Glucose.

Delivery Once the woman's condition has been stabilised, the baby is delivered by the most expedient means. If the woman is not in labour, this usually means caesarean section because induction of labour will take longer.

Postpartum care After delivery, magnesium sulphate infusion is continued for 24 hours and the woman cared for in a high-dependency setting, because the risk of complications takes time to decrease after delivery. Restriction of fluids until diuresis prevents pulmonary oedema. Women with pre-eclampsia are par-

> **Clinical insight**
>
> More pregnant women have epilepsy than eclampsia. In acute clinical situations, it is not always possible to differentiate between the two disorders, because proteinuria is not always present in cases of pre-eclampsia, and epileptic seizure can cause hypertension for a brief period. In cases of doubt, treatment is as for eclampsia.

ticularly vulnerable to this complication due to low oncotic pressure (the ability of blood vessels to retain fluid due to protein content from albumin), endothelial dysfunction and other factors.

6.4 Diabetes

In normal pregnancy, insulin secretion doubles from the end of the first trimester to the end of the third (**Figure 6.2**). This demand cannot be met by the pancreas of a woman with diabetes, or genetic predisposition to diabetes. Therefore, pregnant women with existing, treated diabetes can anticipate increased insulin requirements, and those with gestational diabetes show symptoms by the third trimester.

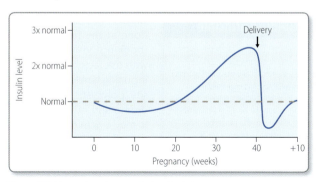

Figure 6.2 Maternal requirements for insulin during pregnancy.

Types

Healthy pregnancy is a prediabetic state of physiological insulin resistance and relative glucose intolerance with the purpose of providing fuel to the fetus. Glucose levels decrease during periods of fasting but increase after a meal.

Diabetes in pregnancy is either gestational or pre-existing.

- **Gestational:** this is a glucose intolerance identified in pregnancy only; it is very likely to recur in the next pregnancy unless the affected woman loses a substantial amount of weight or makes healthy changes to her lifestyle
- **Pre-existing:** this could be type 1 or type 2, and either known before pregnancy or a new presentation

Complications

All types of diabetes in pregnancy put mother and fetus at risk of complications (**Table 6.4**). This is higher for pre-pregnancy diabetes than gestational diabetes.

In labour, there are increased risks of:
- Induction of labour
- Labour dystocia
- Caesarean section
- Instrumental birth
- Perineal trauma
- Shoulder dystocia.

> **Guiding principle**
>
> Type 1 diabetes mellitus rarely presents for the first time in pregnancy. Ketone levels must be assessed in any pregnant woman who is unwell and hyperglycaemic. Ketones indicate that fat catabolism is occurring due to the body's inability to utilise glucose from the blood because of a critical insulin deficiency. If not diagnosed and treated, absolute insulin deficiency leads to maternal death.

Diagnostic approach

Glucose tolerance testing is done at the first antenatal (booking) visit for women with risk factors for diabetes including family history, obesity, polycystic ovarian syndrome and others, because it may uncover previously undetected T2DM. It is also carried out for all women at about 26 weeks (range, 24–28 weeks).

Complications	First trimester	Second and third trimester	Postpartum
Maternal	Type 2 diabetes mellitus (T2DM): ↑ risk of miscarriage	Both T2DM and gestational diabetes: ↑ risk of pregnancy-induced hypertension and pre-eclampsia complications of macrosomia and polyhydramnios (preterm prelabour rupture of membranes, preterm labour, malpresentation, caesarean section) Type 1 and 2: worsening of diabetic retinopathy and nephropathy ↑ insulin requirements	Gestational diabetes: 50% lifetime risk of T2DM
Fetal	Type 1 and type 2 diabetes mellitus: 25% incidence of malformation with HbA1c of >10% = 86 mmol/mol	Both T2DM and gestational diabetes: macrosomia, intrauterine growth restriction, relative hypoxia, polycythaemia, fetal death in utero and stillbirth, ↑ perinatal mortality	Respiratory distress syndrome and transient tachypnoea, hypoglycaemia, polycythaemia, jaundice, metabolic reprogramming leading to ↑ likelihood of obesity and diabetes

Table 6.4 Pre-existing maternal diabetes and gestational diabetes: maternal and fetal complications

To prepare for the test, the woman is asked not to eat anything from the evening before the appointment. A finger-prick blood glucose test is done to check for marked hyperglycaemia, which is diagnostic of diabetes and a contraindication for the glucose tolerance test. If the finger-prick test result is normal, a blood specimen is obtained for measurement of fasting glucose concentration. The woman is then asked to drink a solution containing 75 g of glucose. Blood specimens are drawn 1 and 2 hours later for further measurements of glucose concentration.

A minority of women might have undiagnosed T2DM. Consider the possibility of undiagnosed T2DM as this is associated with poorer outcomes (**Table 6.5**).

Management

Women who share the same type of diabetes cannot be assumed to be at equivalent risk of complications. Excellent control is possible in motivated women with either type 1 or type 2 diabetes mellitus, and gestational diabetes ranges from well controlled by diet to exceedingly poorly controlled and accompanied by many associated complications.

Metformin is considered safe in pregnancy but is not in common use because long-term safety data is not well established. It is used to treat women who have difficulty adhering to insulin therapy and those with T2DM. It delays the need for insulin and decreases total insulin requirements.

Gestational diabetes This is treated initially with lifestyle changes: switching to a diet low in refined sugar and taking

Type of diabetes	Fasting glucose concentration (mmol/L)	1-hour glucose concentration (mmol/L)	2-hour glucose concentration (mmol/L)
Gestational diabetes	≥5.1	≥10.0	≥8.5
Type 2 diabetes mellitus in pregnancy	≥7.0	No value	≥11.1
*Australian Diabetes in Pregnancy Society–International Association of the Diabetes in Pregnancy Study Groups–World Health Organization.			

Table 6.5 Glucose tolerance test: diagnostic criteria for gestational and type 2 diabetes mellitus in pregnancy*

regular exercise. More than three measurements of blood glucose concentration above the target value over a week is generally an indication for starting insulin therapy.

Pre-existing diabetes The care of pregnant women with T2DM is shared with an endocrinologist. Screening for end-organ complications is carried out in each trimester, as well as measurement of glycosylated haemoglobin (HbA1c).

Pregnancies in women with diabetes are considered 'high risk'. Therefore, counselling is available to women with pre-existing diabetes who wish to become pregnant. They are asked about their insulin regimen, known complications, and ophthalmic, renal and podiatry reviews. In addition:
- Oral hypoglycaemic agents and other medications are reviewed, and those known to be teratogenic are substituted with safer options
- High-dose (5 mg) folic acid is prescribed (because of the higher risk of neural tube defects)
- Ultrasound scans are arranged: a dating scan, a 12-week morphology scan and a mid-trimester (morphology) scan at a tertiary centre (because of the increased incidence of cardiac and neurological malformations)

Serial assessments of fetal growth are required after 26–28 weeks.

Delivery In most hospitals, the use of insulin is an indication for delivery by 39 weeks' gestation. Decreasing insulin requirements of up to 10% in late pregnancy is accepted as normal, but any higher suggests impending placental failure and therefore the baby should be delivered. This is planned vaginally with induction of labour if the estimated fetal weight at term is <4.5 kg.

Postpartum care After the birth, paediatric review is required to determine the need for admission to the special neonatal care unit and neonatal blood glucose testing. Maternal glucose concentration is measured four times daily (fasting and 2 hours postprandially) until values become normal without treatment. If maternal blood glucose is persistently high, input from an endocrinologist is required.

6.5 Chorioamnionitis

Chorioamnionitis is inflammation of the chorion and amnion in response to infection of the amniotic fluid. The infection subsequently affects the fetus and mother. Chorioamnionitis is more common in women with PPROM, taking immunosuppressants or with vaginal infections (e.g. bacterial vaginosis, chlamydia, gonorrhoea and other pathogenic organisms). This is because the cause is most commonly an ascending infection from the vagina.

Diagnostic approach

Differential diagnoses, such as urinary tract infection and pneumonia, should be excluded because their treatment does not require delivery. Chorioamnionitis is suspected when a history of fever and flu-like symptoms is combined with uterine pain, contractions or abnormal vaginal discharge. It is unusual to develop chorioamnionitis in the presence of intact membranes. However, the presence of intact membranes does not exclude the diagnosis.

Investigations

Blood specimens are obtained for culture, full blood examination and measurement of inflammatory markers. If a woman appears very unwell, a venous blood gas analysis provides rapid basic information including blood lactate concentration. A septic screen with blood, vaginal and urine culture is required. If pneumonia is suspected, a chest X-ray is carried out.

Management

Chorioamnionitis cannot be treated adequately by antibiotics alone with an ongoing pregnancy, and the uterus needs to be emptied for them to work effectively. Delivery is always indicated, regardless of gestation, because of the significant risk of severe maternal illness and death from sepsis. Chorioamnionitis also carries a significant risk of neonatal morbidity and mortality.

Medication Broad-spectrum IV antibiotic therapy is administered in the same doses as for cases of severe sepsis. Ideally, agents with high placental transfer (e.g. ampicillin) are used, to allow simultaneous treatment of the fetus. Timely intensive care is arranged if there is no response to fluid resuscitation, because inotropic support of the mother's circulation is required in these cases.

Delivery Labour in women with chorioamnionitis is typically more rapid than in non-infected women. However, postpartum haemorrhage is more common.

Postpartum care The placenta is sent for histopathological and microbiological investigation, because the results guide antibiotic therapy for the baby. Administration to the mother of broad-spectrum antibiotics is continued until she is afebrile for 24 hours at minimum. Thereafter, therapy is de-escalated to a course of oral antibiotics.

6.6 Hyperemesis gravidarum

Hyperemesis gravidarum is vomiting that causes weight loss and ketosis and necessitates admission to hospital. It affects about 1% of pregnant women. It is highly likely to recur in subsequent pregnancies.

Management

The condition is treated conservatively in the first instance. Affected women are advised to have adequate rest, consume small, bland meals and eat before rising from bed in the morning. Strict pre-emptive emesis control is key, and this usually requires multiple agents (**Table 6.6**). Thiamine (vitamin B1) supplementation and antacids are given to reduce the risk of Wernicke's encephalopathy (neurological symptoms caused by oxidative damage and impaired glucose metabolism when excessive vomiting leads to depletion of thiamine) and oesophagitis, respectively. By strictly adhering to the antiemetic regimen, women can avoid the need for steroids, which are effective in treating nausea but associated with diabetes, adrenal suppression and osteoporosis. Rarely, all these measures fail and nasogastric or nasojejunal feeding or parenteral nutrition is required.

Medication	Mechanism	Adverse effects or comments
Thiamine (vitamin B1)	Prevention of Wernicke's encephalopathy	Prevents CNS injury and oxidative stress from thiamine deficiency
Pyridoxine (vitamin B6)	Unknown	Often combined with doxylamine
Metoclopramide	Antiemetic: dopamine antagonist	Dystonia, akathisia, idiosyncratic dyskinesia (which may be permanent) Often not very effective
Ondansetron	Antiemetic: 5HT3 antagonist	Effective More expensive Available in orally disintegrating wafer if woman is unable to tolerate tablets Constipation common
Doxylamine	Antiemetic: antihistamine	Sedation, weight gain
Promethazine	Antiemetic: antihistamine	Sedation, weight gain
Prochlorperazine	Antiemetic: antihistamine	Sedation, weight gain
Prednisolone	Steroid: antiemetic via multiple mechanisms	Risks of impaired glucose tolerance, diabetes, adverse lipids, cushingoid habitus, osteopenia and osteoporosis
Multivitamin	Empiric treatment of micronutrient deficiency	Avoid iron, because it exacerbates symptoms
Ranitidine	Antacid: H2 receptor antagonist	Reflux oesophagitis common with recurrent vomiting Proton pump inhibitor may be required

Table 6.6 Hyperemesis: medications used

Fetal growth is monitored with regular (at least monthly) US scans from 26–28 weeks. This is because of the increased risk of intrauterine growth restriction.

Delivery Most women with hyperemesis experience rapid relief from their symptoms once the placenta has been delivered. Therefore, documentation of an agreed gestation at which the baby will be delivered is helpful to the mother's psychological well-being.

> **Guiding principle**
>
> Women with hyperemesis gravidarum are at increased risk of depression. Therefore, psychological support is always offered.

6.7 Acute fatty liver of pregnancy

Acute fatty liver of pregnancy is rare but very serious, affecting roughly 1 in 10,000 pregnancies, usually in the late third trimester. Incidence is increased in:
- Primigravidae
- Multiple pregnancies
- Pregnancies in which the fetus is male
- Women with obesity

The condition is associated with maternal heterozygosity for long-chain 3-hydroxyacyl-coenzyme A dehydrogenase (LCHAD). However, this is rarely known before pregnancy, and screening is not recommended.

Presenting symptoms are frequently non-specific, but the most common are:
- Epigastric or right upper quadrant pain
- Nausea
- Anorexia
- Malaise
- Vomiting and confusion

Examination reveals right upper quadrant tenderness and mild hypertension. Dipstick urinalysis shows proteinuria. Jaundice, if present, excludes pre-eclampsia.

Diagnostic approach

It is often difficult to differentiate AFLP from pre-eclampsia, HELLP syndrome and obstetric cholestasis. Indeed, the pathophysiology underlying these disorders is similar and they may exist along a spectrum. Diagnostic work-up needs to exclude a non-pregnancy-related cause of liver dysfunction, including autoimmune disease, viral hepatitis, medication use and vascular pathology. However, in practice, much of this work is done after the woman's condition has been stabilised and the baby has been delivered.

In suspected cases of AFLP, the work-up is similar to that of pre-eclampsia (see page 142), with the addition of tests to assess synthetic and metabolic liver function (international normalised ratio, blood glucose concentration and ammonia level) and US assessment of the liver (if the clinical situation permits).

Management

The baby is delivered by the most expedient mode of birth once the woman's condition has been stabilised and hypoglycaemia and coagulopathy have been resolved. Care is provided in a high-dependency setting.

6.8 Pulmonary embolism

The risk of venous thromboembolism and subsequent pulmonary embolism is increased from early in the first trimester through to the end of the puerperium (the period after delivery during which the uterus returns to its normal size). Three factors (Virchow's triad) are responsible for this increased risk.

- **Hypercoagulability:** in early pregnancy, there is an oestrogen-mediated increase in procoagulant factors including fibrin and thrombin and a decrease of anti-thrombotic protein S
- **Stasis:** later in pregnancy, venous stasis ensues because of changes to the venous system (e.g. compression of large veins by the gravid uterus)
- **Endothelial injury:** endothelial injury occurs during delivery

The risk of venous thromboembolism increases from 10 per 10,000 woman-years outside pregnancy to 20 in 10,000 during pregnancy and 60 in 10,000 in the puerperium. The risk is doubled if a woman gives birth by caesarean section. However, these numbers are small in absolute terms.

> **Clinical insight**
>
> Measuring the concentration of D-dimer (a marker of blood clot breakdown) is not recommended. A positive result is not confirmatory, because D-dimer is normally increased in pregnancy. Conversely, a negative result does not definitively exclude pulmonary embolism in a woman with symptoms.

Diagnostic approach
A chest X-ray is required to exclude other diagnoses, such as pneumonia. This is typically followed by CT pulmonary angiography or ventilation-perfusion scanning.

Investigations
Haematological findings include neutrophilia and increased C-reactive protein concentration, in addition to hypoxia and hypocarbia on blood gas analysis.

Doppler US is used to assess lower-limb clot burden. CT pulmonary angiography or ventilation-perfusion scanning is needed to visualise the pulmonary embolus itself. However, both techniques require exposure to radiation. Pregnant women with suspected pulmonary embolism who wish to avoid radiation may be offered duplex lower-limb US instead. If a deep vein thrombosis (DVT) is detected, pulmonary embolus is treated on clinical diagnosis. The absence of a lower limb clot means that a CT pulmonary angiography or ventilation-perfusion scan is still required to confirm the diagnosis.

Management
Treatment for pulmonary embolism requires input from a haematologist. Low-molecular-weight heparin, an anticoagulant medication, is given. Compression stockings of the appropriate

> **Clinical insight**
>
> A CT pulmonary angiography study exposes the metabolically active maternal breast to radiation. In 20-year-old women, this causes one additional case of breast cancer for every 143 women scanned. For all women, the lifetime risk of breast cancer is increased by 7%.

> **Clinical insight**
>
> Remember to counsel the woman to avoid oestrogen-containing medications for both contraception after the birth and hormone replacement therapy in future years.

grade are provided. Doppler US is used to assess for residual clot burden in the lower limbs. If the embolus is significant, echocardiography is required at diagnosis to assess cardiac function. Fetal growth is monitored monthly by US. Timed induction of labour or caesarean section at term is advised, because this allows timely adjustment of anticoagulation management to balance the risks of clotting and bleeding during delivery.

An inferior vena cava filter (a device that is inserted into the inferior vena cava to prevent migration of venous thromboemboli into the lungs), inserted in the late third trimester by an interventional radiologist, is clinically useful to reduce further embolus in women at high risk of pulmonary embolism. This group includes women with a very large embolus or significant residual thrombus, who received the diagnosis near term, or who are likely to require a prolonged period of suspension from anticoagulation therapy around the time of delivery.

Once anticoagulation therapy has been discontinued, a screen for inherited and acquired thrombophilias is required. Some types of hormonal contraception are associated with an increased risk of venous thromboembolism. Therefore, women who have had a pulmonary embolism are advised to choose an oestrogen-free contraceptive (e.g. the progestogen-only pill).

6.9 Other maternal diseases during pregnancy

Pregnant women may present with many conditions that, without appropriate management, can lead to complications. They often require input from other medical specialities beyond the pregnancy.

Thyroid dysfunction

Maternal hypothyroidism is associated with lower intelligence quotient (IQ) in the offspring. Hyperthyroidism carries the risk of fetal or neonatal thyrotoxicosis due to transplacental passage of thyroid receptor–stimulating antibodies.

Management

Pregnant women with hypothyroidism require thyroid function tests and a thyroid antibody screen. The dose of levothyroxine (the prescribed form of thyroxine) they receive is increased to anticipate the one-third to one-half increase in thyroxine requirement during pregnancy.

If control of maternal hypothyroidism is poor or there is a risk of fetal thyrotoxicosis (due to maternal hyperthyroidism), fetal growth is assessed by US in the third trimester. Thyroid function tests are required for the neonate, because screening for congenital hypothyroidism (part of the Guthrie test on blood collected by heel prick) is based only on increased concentration of thyroid-stimulating hormone.

Respiratory disease

Asthma poses a risk to the health of the mother and fetus if it is severe or suboptimally controlled. Pregnant women with severe asthma are at risk of severe attacks due to compromise in respiratory mechanics from the pregnancy. The fetus is at risk of intrauterine growth restriction and low birthweight.

Many women stop taking their medications during pregnancy because of concerns about teratogenesis. However, asthma medications, such as the inhaled and short-term oral steroids used to treat exacerbations, are safe for use during pregnancy.

Cardiovascular disease

Cardiovascular disease complicates up to 4% of pregnancies, and heart disease is a leading cause of maternal death in high-income countries. Women with cardiovascular disease are counselled about the pregnancy-associated risks before trying to conceive. Their pregnancies are managed by a multidisciplinary team, and those at high risk of complications are treated in hospitals offering specialised care.

Congenital cardiac disease

In all but minor cases, pregnant women with congenital cardiac disease are cared for by a specialist in maternofetal medicine. The fetus is at a 5% risk of congenital cardiac disease, usually manifesting as a similar lesion to the maternal lesion. A morphology scan carried out in a tertiary centre and a fetal echocardiogram at 24–26 weeks increase the likelihood of antenatal detection. The maternal risk of thrombosis and endocarditis is assessed.

Ischaemic heart disease

Older women are more likely than younger ones to have ischaemic heart disease as, in addition to age, they are more likely to have other risk factors such as smoking, diabetes and obesity. For this reason, acute myocardial infarction is a common indirect cause of maternal death in this population.

Essential hypertension

Essential hypertension, also called chronic hypertension, is a major risk factor for cardiovascular disease and the commonest type of hypertension that women may have had before pregnancy. However, other causes of pre-pregnancy hypertension must be excluded.

The use of angiotensin-converting enzyme inhibitors is ceased, because of their harmful effects on the fetus. A pregnancy-preferred antihypertensive agent, such as labetalol, nifedipine or methyldopa, is used instead. Physiological changes can be expected to reduce antihypertensive requirements in the first and second trimester.

Intrauterine growth restriction is more common in the pregnancies of hypertensive women. Therefore, two or three US assessments of fetal growth are required in the third trimester.

Renal disease

Most renal conditions pose no significant problems in pregnancy. However, the diagnosis requires clarification through directed history taking. because many are heritable. Current renal function is checked, and the woman is assessed for hypertension, renal anaemia, renal stones and infection. A creatinine above 250 μmol/L or renal dialysis is generally a contraindication to pregnancy.

Women with renal disease are asked about previous urinary tract infections; these are common and will require regular screening or antibiotic prophylaxis. They are at increased chance of infection in pregnancy, which, without treatment, is associated with a one-third incidence of pyelonephritis.

Haematological disease

Iron-deficiency anaemia is common in vegetarians, adolescent mothers and women with closely spaced pregnancies. Iron-deficiency anaemia is a risk factor for preterm birth and low birthweight. Therefore, screening is carried out at the first antenatal (booking) visit and at 28 weeks. Treatment is with oral or IV supplementation.

Differential diagnoses for iron-deficiency anaemia include sickle cell disease and thalassaemia, which cause a type of anaemia unrelated to iron levels. In both diseases, the body's ability to produce normal haemoglobin is compromised and the risk of a range of complications is increased. Women who do not have sickle cell disease but who have been identified through screening as carriers of sickle cell trait are offered paternal screening to determine whether the fetus is at risk of sickle cell anaemia (the most serious type of sickle cell disease). Similarly, women identified as carriers of thalassemia trait are offered paternal screening to determine whether the fetus is at risk of major thalassaemia (the most serious type of thalassaemia). If both expectant parents are carriers of either trait, counselling is offered to help them make an informed decision about the chance of their fetus having a major thalassaemia syndrome and the implications of this condition (usually transfusion-dependent anaemia). Specialist input from a haematologist is required.

Gastrointestinal disease

Gastro-oesophageal reflux and peptic ulcer disease are common in both pregnant and non-pregnant women. The main consideration is the safety of the medications used to treat these conditions. Most antacid preparations are safe to use in pregnancy, as are H_2 receptor antagonists and most proton pump inhibitors. Although some clinicians avoid the use of omeprazole in the first trimester, recent data suggest that it is no less safe.

Inflammatory bowel disease

Women with inflammatory bowel disease are asked about the degree to which it is controlled, the use of steroids and biological agents, prior surgery, and known fistulae or perianal disease. Some medications are teratogenic and contraindicated in pregnancy. Long-term steroid use requires additional steroid cover during surgery to prevent an adrenal crisis (due to insufficient levels of endogenous cortisol). In cases of perianal disease, caesarean section is usually recommended for delivery. In Crohn's disease, investigations are required to detect anaemia, which may be due to iron deficiency, vitamin B_{12} deficiency or anaemia of chronic disease.

Monitoring and interventions in labour

chapter 7

7.1 Clinical scenario

Jane, a 31-year-old primigravida, presents in spontaneous labour at 37^{+5} weeks. Her membranes have ruptured and she has thick meconium liquor. She is having four strong contractions every 10 minutes lasting 45–60 seconds each. A cardiotocograph (CTG) is applied. This demonstrated the contractions assessed on uterine palpation (also called 'timing' of contractions). It also shows that the baby has a baseline tachycardia with reduced variability and late decelerations. A vaginal examination is performed and her cervix is 3 cm dilated, 1 cm long, soft with the station at –3. An urgent caesarean section is arranged.

7.2 Abnormal cardiotocograph

Cardiotocography (see page 40) is used to monitor fetal condition during labour if risk factors for fetal compromise are present. Intermittent auscultation of the fetal heart is preferred for women without risk factors, because of the significant incidence of abnormal patterns on a CTG that are false positives for fetal compromise.

There are multiple parameters in a CTG (**Table 7.1**). The greater the abnormal number, the greater the likelihood of fetal hypoxia and true compromise.

Abnormal baseline fetal heart rate

The normal baseline fetal heart rate is 110–160 beats per minute. It is measured in the absence of contractions and fetal movement.

Finding	Common cause	Physiological or pathological changes
Baseline bradycardia	Low inherent baseline	Mature parasympathetic system or input into fetal CRC Idiopathic
	Maternal opiate use	Fetal CRC depression, increased parasympathetic tone
	Fetal arrhythmia	Intermittent or permanent fetal atrioventricular block due to structural cardiac disease or fetal supraventricular tachycardia, usually idiopathic *anti-Ro or *anti-La antibodies
Baseline tachycardia	Maternal fever (infection, epidural, other)	Increased oxygen demands and CO_2 production due to metabolic load of higher temperature
	Fetal infection	Metabolic demands of infection
	Recovery from recent acute hypoxic insult	Physiological response to clear accumulated metabolic byproducts of anaerobic metabolism
Reduced variability	Fetal sleep Fetal sedation	Decreased CRC activity
Absent variability	Fetal hypoxia Heavy fetal sedation	Suppressed fetal CRC with monotonous autonomic tone
Excessive variability	Fetal hypoxia Fetal cord compression	Baroreceptor or chemoreceptor stimulation from hypoxia or wide variation in cord compression and fetal blood pressure
Early deceleration	Fetal head compression Physiological	Vagal stimulation → lowered sinoatrial node firing
Variable deceleration	Umbilical cord compression	Cord occlusion with contraction → hypertension → baroreceptor stimulation → deceleration → removal of cord compression → restoration of fetal heart rate

Table 7.1 Abnormal cardiotocographic patterns: physiological and pathological changes. *Continues opposite*

Finding	Common cause	Physiological or pathological changes
Prolonged deceleration	Tonic contraction	Reduced oxygenated blood from placenta → deceleration in fetal heart rate to reduce oxygen demands, myocardial acidosis and depression, and cerebral anoxia
Late deceleration	Undetected placental failure or intrauterine growth restriction combined with labour contractions	Hypoxic and acidotic fetus with depressed CRC and myocardium unable to mount a normal physiological response to contractions

CRC, cardioregulatory centre.
*anti-Ro and anti-La are maternally produced antibodies that are able to cross the placenta and cause permanent fetal heart block. Women with autoimmune conditions are screened for anti-Ro and anti-La in pregnancy.

Table 7.1 *Continued*

The main baseline abnormalities are:
- Baseline bradycardias (<110 beats per minute)
- Tachycardias (>160 beats per minute)

Baseline bradycardia

> **Clinical insight**
>
> The fetus responds to the maternal environment. Therefore, basic intrauterine resuscitation (as in obstetric emergency management sections below) involves optimising placental perfusion by altering maternal physiological dynamics.

Baseline bradycardia of 100–110 beats per minute is most commonly a finding in fetuses >41 weeks' gestation or during labour when the mother has received parenteral opiates for analgesia (**Figure 7.1**). In these settings and in the absence of other abnormal cardiotocographic findings, it is no reason for concern about fetal wellbeing but CTG is maintained.

The major abnormal causes of this pattern are:
- **Fetal cardiac conduction abnormalities:** the fetal heart rate is often even lower and switches between normal and bradycardic rates

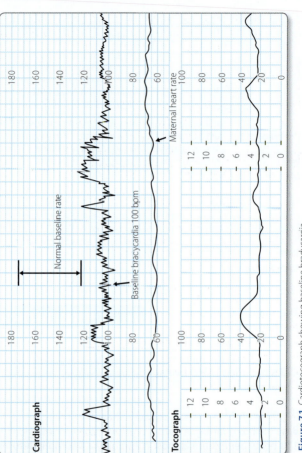

Figure 7.1 Cardiotocograph showing baseline bradycarcia.

- **Decelerations related to hypoxia:** there are usually other abnormal features, an inciting stimulus, and a previously normal baseline heart rate

Baseline tachycardia

Baseline tachycardia (**Figure 7.2**) is more concerning than baseline bradycardia, because possible causes include maternal or fetal infection and fetal hypoxia. Isolated mild tachycardia (160–170 beats per minute) does not indicate compromise. However, because the fetus is at risk of exhausting its physiological reserves if the condition is sustained, and is at risk of deterioration, CTG is continued.

Abnormal variability

Fetal heart rate variability is the deviation from the baseline in number of beats per minute. The abnormal patterns of variability are:
- Reduced variability (3–5 beats per minute)
- Absent variability (<3 beats per minute)
- Excessive variability (>25 beats per minute)

Reduced variability

Reduced variability is a finding in fetal sleep phase and with maternal antihypertensive use or opiate analgesia. In the absence of other abnormalities, no specific action is required.

Absent variability

This is more concerning for hypoxia and rarely occurs in isolation. However, it is occasionally provoked by the same factors that cause reduced variability. Other signs of fetal compromise need to be sought, such as late and prolonged decelerations, because this pattern requires urgent reversal of provocative factors, intrauterine resuscitation (by means of stopping contractions, supporting maternal blood pressure and placental perfusion with intravenous fluid bolus and use of left lateral positioning to remove aortocaval compression) and, potentially, delivery.

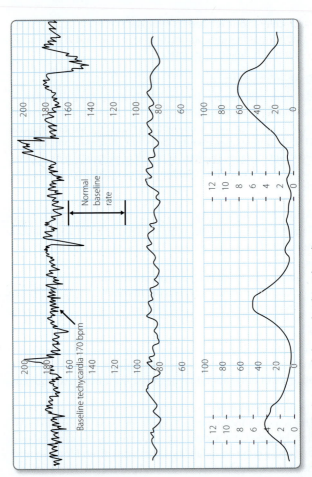

Figure 7.2 Cardiotocograph showing baseline tachycardia.

Excessive variability

This is an uncommon pattern that indicates hypoxia or cord compression. The problem is resolved by removing provocative factors, e.g. by adjusting the dosage of synthetic oxytocin to stop excessive contractions.

Accelerations

An acceleration of fetal heart rate is defined as an increase from baseline of at least 15 beats per minute for 15 seconds or more (**Figure 2.10**). Outside labour, a cardiotocograph showing two accelerations in a 20-minute period in wake phase is normal. During labour, absence of accelerations (with no other abnormal features) is occasionally caused by the physiological challenge of contractions meaning the fetus does not expend excess energy on heart rate acceleration behaviour. Therefore, unless accompanied by other abnormal cardiotocographic features, it is not concerning.

The presence of accelerations is reassuring, especially if there is an abnormal feature such as reduced variability or abnormal baseline heart rate. Accelerations indicate that the fetus has good reserves and is non-hypoxic, and the significance of this finding overrides any concern arising from the presence of the abnormal feature.

Decelerations

The four types of deceleration are:
- Early
- Variable
- Prolonged
- Late

Early decelerations

Early decelerations mirror contractions; each beginning when the contraction begins and ending when it ends (**Figure 7.3**). They are shallow (within a range of about 10–20 beats per minute) and typically occur during fetal sleep phase and when cervical dilatation is 4–8 cm. They are benign and a response to fetal parasympathetic stimulation caused by head compression.

172 Monitoring and interventions in labour

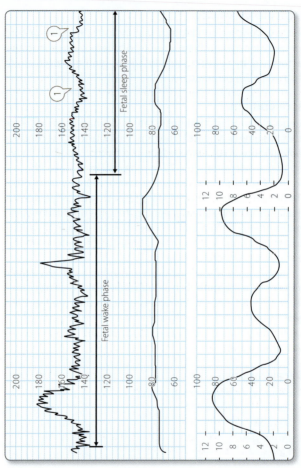

Figure 7.3 Cardiotocograph showing early decelerations: the fetus enters sleep phase and early decelerations mirror contractions.

Variable decelerations

Variable decelerations are variable in terms of timing, depth and shape but generally appear as sharp dips on CTG (**Figure 7.4**). They represent the response of the fetal heart to compression of the umbilical cord during labour and therefore commonly occur with a contraction. 'Shouldering' is the term for the increases in fetal heart rate that are often apparent before and after the deceleration.

- **Simple variable decelerations** are not accompanied by any other abnormal features. They do not indicate fetal compromise
- **Complicated variable decelerations** are variable decelerations associated with another abnormal feature (e.g. slow recovery). They usually indicate subacute fetal hypoxia

Prolonged decelerations

Prolonged decelerations last longer than 90 seconds (**Figure 7.5**). If they extend to 5 minutes, they are termed as bradycardia.

This pattern indicates ongoing acute hypoxia, generally due to one or more of the following:

> **Guiding principle**
>
> Early and variable decelerations are physiological responses to head compression and cord compression, respectively. Although they are abnormal features, neither early nor simple variable decelerations indicate compromise; rather, they are signs of the ability of a well-oxygenated fetus to respond to changes in the intrauterine environment.

- Poor fetal reserve (as a result of intrauterine growth restriction) and contractions
- Uterine hyperstimulation more than five contractions in a 10-minute period or <90 seconds between contractions)
- Maternal hypotension and associated insufficient placental perfusion
- Placental abruption
- Cord prolapse
- Uterine rupture

When prolonged decelerations are present, prompt action is required to resolve any underlying problem (see page 176). However, in the absence of intrauterine growth restriction or a major complication (i.e. placental abruption, cord prolapse or

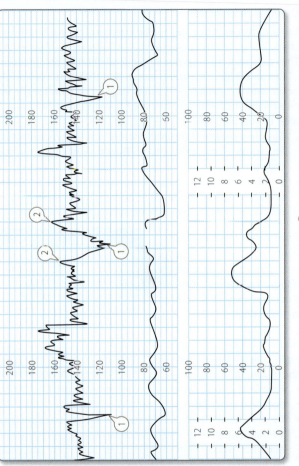

Figure 7.4 Cardiotocograph showing variable decelerations (1), represented by the sharp dips. An increase in fetal heart rate ('shouldering') (2) is also apparent on either side of the deceleration.

Abnormal cardiotocograph

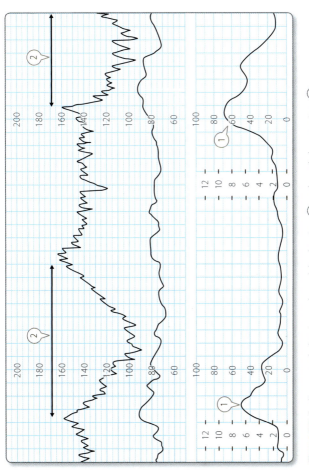

Figure 7.5 Cardiotocograph showing prolonged decelerations (2) and coupled contractions (1).

> **Clinical insight**
>
> If the mother has normal oxygen saturation, there is minimal scope for further oxygenation of the maternal blood. Therefore, provision of oxygen via face mask has little, if any, benefit for the fetus. However, it is useful for preoxygenation if urgent caesarean section under general anaesthesia becomes necessary. Similarly in a normotensive well hydrated woman, intravenous fluids are unlikely to improve fetal status.

uterine rupture), over 90% of cases of prolonged decelerations resolve with conservative measures.

Management is directed at intrauterine resuscitation measures. Call for assistance and halt any oxytocin infusion. Place the mother in the left lateral position to optimise placental perfusion. If low maternal blood pressure is a possibility (e.g. when epidural anaesthesia has been used), administer an intravenous fluid bolus.

In cases of uterine hyperstimulation, terbutaline (see page 129) is used to produce acute tocolysis. The inhibition of contractions gives the fetus opportunity to recover from hypoxia, thereby gaining time for surgery to be arranged or avoiding the need to proceed to immediate birth altogether.

Next, a vaginal examination is carried out. The four aims are:
- To assess the progress of labour and the possibility of vaginal delivery
- To rupture the membranes and assess for meconium-stained liquor. Fetal anal sphincter relaxation and passage of meconium occurs under conditions of acute hypoxia. Furthermore, a hypoxic fetus can gasp in utero, inhaling meconium which leads to plugging of the alveoli (meconium aspiration syndrome)
- To place a fetal scalp electrode, a small metal wire that directly detects fetal heart rate when inserted a few millimetres into the fetal scalp (if maternal serology is negative for HIV or hepatitis – transmission is increased as the technique involves fetal skin breach), to confirm that the heart rate is not maternal
- To assess for fetal reactivity to examination, because a well-oxygenated fetus responds to digital stimulation of the scalp with an acceleration

Late decelerations

Late decelerations start during a contraction but peak afterwards (**Figure 7.6**). They are pathological, indicating significant hypoxia. Urgent delivery is needed, by the most expedient route.

What distinguishes late decelerations from early decelerations is that they start and recover after the contraction has started and stopped, respectively; they do not mirror contractions; and they recur with every contraction ('lates have mates').

> **Clinical insight**
>
> Subtle and shallow decelerations, which are often difficult to spot, are signs of a severely chronically hypoxic fetus with no ability to respond appropriately. They accompany an otherwise 'flat' unreactive CTG and you should look carefully for this pattern when such a CTG is encountered.

7.3 Induction and augmentation of labour

Induction is the process of starting labour artificially. It is used when the risks of continuing pregnancy outweigh the risks of delivery (**Table 7.2**). Even in healthy pregnancies, continuing beyond 39 weeks confers no fetal benefit, and the risk of perinatal mortality increases after this point. Therefore, the indications for induction have low thresholds beyond this gestation.

Augmentation refers to enhancing contractions in a labour that has already commenced spontaneously if a woman's spontaneous contractions are inadequate to achieve cervical dilation.

The methods for induction and augmentation are the same, as both involve uterine stimulation.

Cervical ripening

Induction is more likely to be successful if the cervix is open and the membranes ruptured, because contractions are then more effective. If the cervix is not sufficiently open to rupture the membranes easily, then it has to be made open, i.e. 'ripened'. Options to stimulate cervical ripening are:
- Pharmacological: prostaglandins

178 Monitoring and interventions in labour

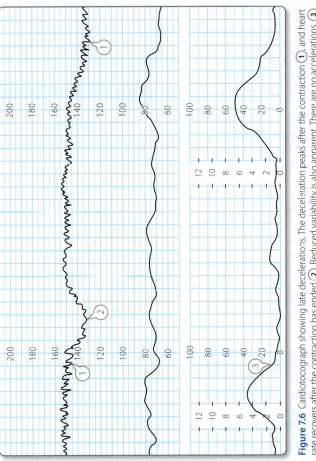

Figure 7.6 Cardiotocograph showing late decelerations. The deceleration peaks after the contraction ①, and heart rate recovers after the contraction has ended ②. Reduced variability is also apparent. There are no accelerations. ③ End of contraction.

Category	Indications
Maternal	Maternal disease Maternal request
Fetal	Intrauterine growth restriction Macrosomia (in selected cases) Decreased movements Abnormal monitoring
Pregnancy	Post-dates pregnancy Hypertension Pre-eclampsia Gestational diabetes

Table 7.2 Induction of labour: indications

- Mechanical:
  - Cervical membrane sweeping
  - Balloon catheter insertion

Prostaglandins and balloon techniques are equally effective, but have different indications and contraindications.

After the cervix is open and membranes ruptured, oxytocin infusion can be used to stimulate contractions.

Cervical membrane sweep

This is a low-risk method for inducing labour. It is offered to all women whose pregnancies have reached 40 weeks. A finger is passed through the cervix and rotated just inside the lower segment of the uterus. This stimulates the release of prostaglandins, which ripen the cervix and stimulate contractions. It decreases the risk of requiring formal mechanical or pharmacological induction and is safe.

Prostaglandins (Table 7.3)

Prostaglandins act by ripening the cervix and stimulating contractions. They are available orally but this is not used for induction of labour, rather they are inserted in the upper vagina in gel or pessary form.

Prostaglandins are helpful when the fetal head is not well engaged in the pelvis as they stimulate uterine activity which

Method	Mechanisms of action	Benefits	Risks
Prostaglandin gel (e.g. dinoprostone, Prostin E2)	Interleukin release Inflammatory infiltrate Remodelling of cervical extracellular matrix	6-hourly dosing Time-efficient	Gel cannot be removed Uterine hyperstimulation requiring emergency caesarean
Prostaglandin pessary (e.g. Cervidil, Misodel)		Easily removed if hyperstimulation occurs Rapid wash-out of effect	Uterine hyperstimulation requiring emergency caesarean
*Both are effective if the fetal head is high, because they stimulate uterine activity that aids descent.			

Table 7.3 Comparison of prostaglandins used to ripen the cervix*

acts to fix the head in the pelvis. They are contraindicated when a uterine scar exists (e.g. previous caesarean) because they create an unacceptable risk of uterine rupture by softening the scar which allows it to tear with contractions.

Balloon catheter insertion (Table 7.4)

This technique is safe to use for nearly all women and is particularly useful where prostaglandins are contraindicated (including prior caesarean section, intrauterine growth restriction and lack of overnight rapid access to caesarean section) as it will not weaken any caesarean section scar and does not cause contractions. The balloon catheter is passed through the external and internal cervical os and then inflated, compressing the cervix and stimulating local remodeling. It is usually left in for >12 hours before being removed.

Artificial rupture of the membranes

If the cervix is already ripe, or once ripening has occurred with one of the above methods, labour may be induced by

Method	Mechanism	Benefits	Risks
Cervical balloon (e.g. Cook, Attard)	Mechanical compression of cervix between two balloons Release of prostaglandins Breakdown of collagen cross-linking Softening and opening	Minimal uterine hyperstimulation risk, so safest for fetuses with intrauterine growth restriction	Pushes high fetal head out of pelvis, causing cord prolapse with artificial rupture of membranes
Foley catheter	Mechanical compression from one balloon above the internal cervical os, then as above		Rupture Need for reinsertion

*Both methods have similar effectiveness.

Table 7.4 Mechanical induction of cervical ripening: comparison of balloon and catheter methods*

rupturing the membranes. This is called 'artificial rupture of the membranes' (ARM). While the membranes are held tense between the examiner's fingers (avoiding the pain-sensitive cervix), an amniotic membrane perforator (e.g. Amnihook) or similar device is used to perforate the membranes with a quick stroke (**Figure 7.7**).

Oxytocin infusion

An oxytocin infusion is used to stimulate contractions to induce labour that has not yet begun, or augment labour that is not progressing adequately. Oxytocin is indicated if spontaneous contractions:
- Prove ineffective, i.e. effect no cervical change, or
- Are inadequate, i.e. are not strong enough to be considered labour contractions, and effect inadequate cervical change

These situations are particularly common in primigravid labours.

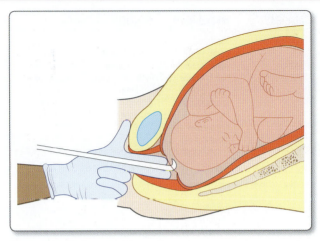

Figure 7.7 Artificial rupture of the membranes.

> ### Guiding principle
> The primigravid and multiparous uterus behave very differently. The primigravid uterus is inefficient and prone to inertia. The multiparous uterus is more forceful and at risk of rupture in efforts to overcome obstruction, particularly in cases of augmented labour. A useful aide-memoire for students is 'Never augment a multiparous uterus', because this is done only under the supervision of a senior colleague and with careful assessment to exclude any sign of obstruction. Lack of progress is more likely due to obstruction than inadequate contractions in a multiparous woman.

Oxytocin is given intravenously at low-dose rates that vary by local protocol and are increased steadily every 30 minutes until three or four contractions occur every 10 minutes.

Adverse effects Increased contraction pain, nausea and vomiting are common adverse effects of oxytocin infusion. The risk of postpartum haemorrhage (PPH) is also higher than in non-augmented labours. Therefore, additional prophylaxis for PPH is considered in the third stage of labour (e.g. ergotamine intramuscular injection, rectal misoprostol or prophylactic oxytocin infusion).

Procedure for induction of labour

The key steps in planning an induction of labour are as follows:
- Determine the indication and urgency: does induction need to occur today, tomorrow or at another time that is convenient for both the mother and the health professionals providing her care?
- Exclude contraindications, such as placenta praevia or non-cephalic lie
- Choose the mode of induction: consider the clinical situation and the favourability of the cervix (see page 29, Table 2.1).

For each of these steps, the findings of abdominal and vaginal examinations are invaluable.

Abdominal examination

Perform an abdominal examination to confirm fetal lie, presentation and station (see page 26). A non-cephalic lie or an unengaged head presentation both require active management and preclude routine induction. For example, a breech presentation is managed with external cephalic version (see page 122) or caesarean section rather than induction.

If the head is not engaged, the risk of cord prolapse is increased. If induction is unavoidable, the membranes are ruptured only by an experienced clinician, ideally in the presence of contractions and with stabilisation of the fetal position, with manual abdominal pressure to maintain the vertex over the cervix.

Vaginal examination

Cervical favourability is assessed by vaginal examination and Bishop scoring (see page 29).

Favourable cervix Favourability of the cervix improves the likelihood that an induction of labour will result in a vaginal birth. A favourable cervix implies the one that is soft and slightly open and this is standardised by means of Bishop scoring. Women with a Bishop's score of 6 or more are offered induction with simultaneous artificial rupture of membranes and oxytocin infusion. If a woman has a history of fast labours or grand multiparity

> **Clinical insight**
>
> Sensitive examinations are always carried out in a manner that maintains a woman's dignity. A chaperone is provided, if required, and the curtains are drawn. The woman is given privacy to undress and dress alone, and she is provided with a sheet to cover areas that are not being examined. The experience is less uncomfortable for the woman if the examination jelly is first warmed by the examiner's gloved hands.

(five or more children), or wishes to wait, an interval of several hours before the start of oxytocin infusion is acceptable, because artificial rupture of membranes alone usually causes spontaneous labour contractions.

Unfavourable cervix An unfavourable cervix is firm and closed and not prepared for labour. This is formalised by the use of Bishop scoring. For women with a Bishop's score below 6, the choice is between mechanical and pharmacological cervical ripening depending on clinical factors (see page 179). After the cervix has been made favourable, management proceeds as for a favourable cervix.

Intrapartum care

Before induction begins, an intravenous (IV) cannula (18-gauge or above allowing faster flow of intravenous fluids than smaller cannulae is prudent given the potential for postpartum haemorrhage) is placed in the dorsum of the woman's non-dominant hand. The cardiotocograph is checked, because it must be normal to proceed safely, and should be continued as contractions are being artificially stimulated. It is confirmed that the woman's bladder has recently been emptied and that she understands the process.

Cardiotocographic monitoring is maintained throughout the induction. As in spontaneous labour, 4-hourly abdominal and vaginal examinations are carried out to assess progress. The first of these takes place approximately 4 hours after the diagnosis of active labour.

Anaesthesia Labour is a painful process and many women experience induced and augmented contractions more painfully than spontaneous ones. Pain and anxiety cause elevated catecholamines and this contributes to stalled labour as they counteract the effects of oxytocin. For this reason, women who are augmented for slow progress are offered a medically indicated epidural. Epidural anaesthesia encourages relaxation, and lowers the levels of circulating maternal catecholamines released in response to stress.

> **Clinical insight**
>
> Wide-bore intravenous access is preferred in labouring women, because of the risk of PPH, which can be both rapid and profuse. The antecubital fossa (the anterior elbow) is avoided to ensure that the line does not become kinked repeatedly as the woman labours and moves her arm spontaneously.

7.4 Instrumental delivery

In an instrumental (also termed 'operative' or 'assisted') vaginal delivery, the accoucheur facilitates delivery of the fetus, most commonly with the use of a vacuum extractor or forceps. Common indications for this mode of delivery are listed in **Table 7.5**. About 15% of vaginal births are instrumental deliveries.

The prerequisites for instrumental delivery are listed in the 'FORCEPS' mnemonic.
- **F:** Fully dilated cervix
- **O:** Occipitoanterior position Or position known (and ability to rotate)
- **R:** Ruptured membranes
- **C:** Consent, Catheter or bladder emptied
- **E:** Engaged head (i.e. in a safe position for vaginal delivery to be attempted; see page 83)
- **P:** Pain relief
- **S:** Adequate pelvic Space, Scissors for episiotomy and consider Shoulders Sticking (shoulder dystocia)

For various reasons, the use of epidural anaesthesia has increased over the past few

> **Guiding principle**
>
> After any difficult or emergency delivery, the woman and her partner are debriefed by the accoucheur in the days after the birth. A significant proportion (1:20) of women who have an instrumental birth meet criteria for acute post-traumatic stress response and can consequently defer or choose not to have a subsequent pregnancy. For this reason, giving clear explanations of the procedure to the woman and encouraging her to be actively involved during the birth, respecting her wishes, documenting events, providing adequate pain relief and debriefing are essential.

Maternal	Fetal	Labour
Unable to push Neuromuscular weakness Spinal cord injury	Non-reassuring cardiotocograph in second stage	Prolonged second stage with inadequate progress and maternal exhaustion
Should not push CNS pathology: aneurysm, increased intracranial pressure, recent stroke Cardiovascular pathology: aortic aneurysm or dilatation, cardiac or valvular disease, connective tissue disease affecting great vessels		

Table 7.5 Instrumental birth: indications

decades. This has been accompanied by an increase in the need for instrumental delivery, because women who receive an epidural have difficulty feeling their contractions, and also 'push' less effectively due to loss of afferent sensory input.

Rates of instrumental delivery are reduced by:
- Active labour positioning in upright postures
- Use of oxytocin infusion in nulliparae to optimise contractions and correct malposition by encouraging the fetal head to rotate and fit maternal pelvic dimensions
- Manual rotation of the fetal head by the examining obstetrician to the occipitoanterior position at the end of the first stage of labour
- Allowance for 1 hour of passive descent when epidural anaesthesia is present before commencing active second stage 'pushing'
- If mother and baby are well, prolongation of an active second stage beyond 2 hours for nulliparae and 1 hour for multiparae

Classification

Instrumental births are classified by the fetal station (see chapter 4) and the presence or absence of rotation to the occipitoanterior position.
- **Midcavity:** vaginally at ischial spines to +2 station and less than one-fifth palpable or no head abdominally

- **Low:** below +2 station vaginally, visible with pushing and not palpable abdominally
- **Outlet:** visible without spreading the labia, a presenting part this low is within 45° of the midline (usually occipitoanterior but occasionally occipitoposterior), because this dimension accommodates the maternal pelvic outlet. If another position is found (e.g. occipitotransverse), either the station is overestimated due to caput succedaneum (swelling on the presenting part of the fetal head) or the position is incorrect
- **Rotational:** with rotation beyond 45° from the midline

Instruments

The two major instruments used to assist in delivery are the vacuum extractor and forceps. Choosing the correct one is key to minimising the risk of harm to the baby, because if two instruments are used sequentially, the individual risks of each instrument are additive. The choice of instrument depends on operator experience and preference, maternal status (effectiveness of maternal effort, analgesia, perineal flexibility) and fetal position.

In any case of doubt about which instrument to use to assist the birth or suitability for assisted birth, the assistance of a senior colleague is sought and the woman is transferred to the operating theatre and the birth is assisted in an environment where a caesarean section can be carried out, if assisted vaginal birth fails. This reduces the risk of the accoucheur applying excess traction and causing fetal harm.

Vacuum extractor

A vacuum extractor (also known as a ventouse) is a cup-shaped device attached to a mechanism providing suction (**Figure 7.8**). The application of negative pressure to the fetal scalp sucks fetal tissue into the margin of the cup; this provides the lever for applied traction. **Table 7.6** summarises the advantages and disadvantages of vacuum-assisted delivery.

Infants delivered by this method have a 'chignon' of tissue and fluid from the effects of negative pressure on the scalp. The parents are reassured that it will disappear within a day or two.

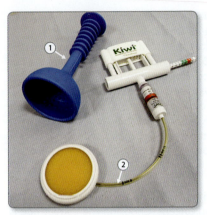

Figure 7.8 Vacuum extractor. (1) Silastic cup; (2) Omni cup (Kiwi™).

Advantages	Disadvantages
Decreased requirement for maternal analgesia Lower risk of maternal pelvic floor and perineal trauma Non-occipitoanterior presentations can be autorotated, in the optimal position in the maternal pelvis, to the occipitoanterior position for vaginal delivery	Failure rate higher than for forceps; generally, the station needs to be lower and maternal effort greater than that with forceps Difficult application, with extensive caput succedaneum and moulding Relies on optimal positioning for the fetal head to be guided past the narrowest diameters of the maternal pelvis; without it, the failure rate is high Greater fetal scalp trauma, cephalohaematoma, subgaleal haematoma (which can cause life-threatening neonatal cardiovascular collapse due to the size of the potential space) Contraindicated in cases of gestation <34 weeks, non-vertex presentation, suspected fetal bleeding disorder

Table 7.6 Instrumental delivery with a vacuum extractor: advantages and disadvantages

Forceps

Different types of forceps are available for different types of birth (**Figure 7.9**). All have shanks, a locking mechanism and a

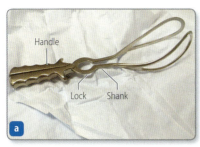

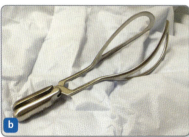

Figure 7.9 Obstetric forceps. (a) Neville-Barnes forceps. Note the long handle for leverage and the pelvic curve. (b) Wrigley's forceps. Note the short handle, suitable for caesarean sections. Rhodes forceps are also used and are very similar.

cephalic curve to accommodate the fetal head. Forceps designed for occipitoanterior births also have a pelvic curve to accommodate the maternal pelvis; an example is the Neville-Barnes (see **Figure 7.9a**). In contrast, forceps used to rotate a non-occipitoanterior presentation do not have this curve, because it would injure the maternal pelvis during rotation.

> **Clinical insight**
>
> Babies born by instrumental delivery are not given hats, because surveillance for subperiosteal and intracranial bleeding is required; in rare cases, these lead to cephalohaematoma and subgaleal haematoma, respectively. The mother is advised to inform staff if she has any concerns about her baby.

The Neville-Barnes forceps are one of the most common types of forceps encountered. They are used for non-rotational birth.

Advantages The advantages of forceps lie in their ability to speedily effect delivery when necessary, with little or no reliance on maternal effort and with a low chance of failure.

Forceps are the instrument of choice in cases of prematurity of <34 weeks, when maternal expulsive efforts are contraindicated, and in cases of after-coming head of the breech or face presentation. Forceps are preferred to vacuum extraction in cases of significant caput and moulding. They are also appropriate when vacuum failure occurs and the head is at the pelvic outlet.

Disadvantages The use of forceps carries the following risks, which are related to their mechanism of action.
- Increased risk of trauma to the maternal pelvic floor and perineum
- Neonatal marks, bruising and rarely facial nerve trauma
- Greater requirement for procedural analgesia

They are also subject to various limitations, such as the inability to apply non-rotational forceps unless the head is close to directly occipitoanterior (or posterior). Considerable procedural skill is required, particularly for rotational forceps use.

Procedure

Assisted vaginal birth requires careful assessment of the labour progress and, in particular, the anticipated success of the procedure to ensure it is appropriate. Complications are significantly more probable for failed instrumental births, particularly, when they are conducted in an operating theatre by junior staff. Anticipating common complications such as shoulder dystocia and postpartum haemorrhage allows preventative action and reduces their severity.

History

Enquiries are made to determine:
- Gestation, progress of labour and how oxytocin has been used to augment labour
- Estimated size of the fetus, and its last known position and station
- Cardiotocographic results and liquor status (presence of meconium)

If instrumental delivery is indicated, verbal or written consent is obtained. A midwife must be present to care for the mother.

A paediatrician, second midwife and resuscitaire also attend to care for the baby. Forceps, episiotomy scissors, cord clamps, a third-stage uterotonic agent (such as oxytocin or ergometrine, or a combination of both) and a perineal repair kit are needed.

Examination

Both of the following are used to confirm that instrumental delivery is appropriate. If these conditions are not met, caesarean section should be arranged.

- **Abdominal examination:** this is needed to determine fetal station in fifths (the presenting part should not be palpable) and the side of the fetal back (this helps establish vaginal position)
- **Vaginal examination:** this is done to assess cervical dilation (the cervix should be fully dilated), fetal position, station, caput and moulding.

Vacuum extractor technique

The woman is placed in the lithotomy position, with a hip wedge. Her buttocks are moved to the edge of the bed, and her bladder is emptied by catheter. Pillows placed under her head encourage maternal participation by allowing her to observe the birth. The following steps are then carried out:

- If episiotomy is likely to be needed, e.g. for primigravidae and in cases of rigid perineum or rapid delivery, the site is infiltrated with local anaesthetic; it requires time to take effect
- With the labia parted, the cup is inserted between contractions to the flexion point, 3 cm anterior to the posterior fontanelle. A finger is used to check that no maternal tissues are included. Full suction is then applied. One finger is placed on the fetal scalp and a thumb on the cup to ensure that descent occurs with traction (**Figure 7.10**)
- Traction (in line with the cup) is applied simultaneously with maternal effort
- An episiotomy is made, if needed. As the head crowns, the maternal perineum is protected with the hand that is not delivering the baby. On delivery, the baby is placed on the mother's chest

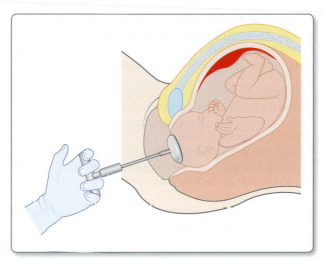

Figure 7.10 Vacuum extractor technique. An occipitoposterior fetus has a cup applied. Then traction over successive contractions elicits descent and rotation to occipitoanterior in the portion of the maternal pelvis where this is naturally able to occur.

> **Clinical insight**
>
> Generally, no more than three contractions are required to effect delivery with the help of a vacuum extractor. Unless birth is imminent or other significant manoeuvres have been carried out, abandoning vacuum-assisted delivery for caesarean section or completing delivery with the use of forceps is safer than persisting. If descent and rotation to the occipitoanterior position from non-occipitoanterior have been carried out, up to six total contractions may be required.

The remainder of the birth is completed as in an uncomplicated vaginal birth (see page 81).

Forceps technique

Positioning is as for vacuum extraction, but the maternal requirement for analgesia is greater. If the woman does not have effective epidural anaesthesia, a pudendal block is given and allowed time to take effect.

The following procedure describes the use of non-rotational forceps (e.g. Neville-Barnes) for an occipitoanterior or a posterior presentation.

- The forceps are assembled. They must lock and be in the position in which they will be applied to the fetal head ('ghost application'). The blades are covered with obstetric cream for lubrication. The right blade is placed within easy reach on the delivery table
- The left blade, held in the left hand, is inserted into the posterior aspect of the vagina, where the sacral hollow provides space for the manoeuvre. The maternal tissues are simultaneously protected with the right hand. The left blade is always inserted first, regardless of the handedness of the accoucheur, due to the direction of the locking mechanism

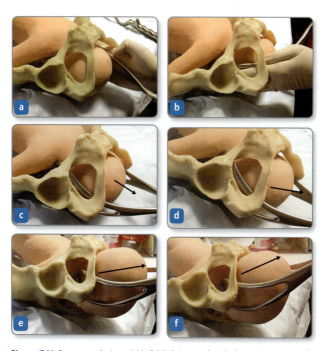

Figure 7.11 Forceps technique. (a) Left blade inserted, with the vagina protected. (b) Right blade inserted, mirroring the left and locked. (c) Initial traction vector inferiorly following the maternal pelvis. (d) Blades gently raised as the occiput clears the symphysis. (e) Blades raised further as the occiput clears the symphysis. (f) Blades elevated to deliver the face.

> **Clinical insight**
>
> Compared with non-instrumental vaginal delivery, forceps delivery carries a higher risk of perineal trauma, because the forceps increase the presenting diameter. For this reason, episiotomy is almost always necessary. Once delivery is inevitable, disarticulating the forceps on the perineum with crowning reduces the risk of trauma by reducing stretching of the tissue.

- The forceps is guided gently across the maternal thigh in an arc, so that the blade comes to lie alongside the fetal head and ear (**Figure 7.11a**)
- The right blade is used to perform the same manoeuvre as for the left blade but on the opposite side (**Figure 7.11b**). The blades should lock easily
- A check is carried out to ensure that the blades are aligned correctly, with the sagittal suture midway between them. The forceps are then used to pull down the fetal head with each maternal contraction, in the same arc as for vacuum-assisted delivery (**Figures 7.11c to 7.11f**)
- An episiotomy (a surgical incision to enlarge the introitus made at a 60° angle away from the anus) is made when the head is crowning. Delivery is then completed

7.5 Caesarean section

Caesarean section is the surgical procedure by which a baby is delivered via an incision made through the mother's abdomen and uterus. In the UK, about 25–30% of all deliveries are via caesarean section.

Caesarean sections are termed as elective if the procedure is planned to take place at a specific time. All other caesarean sections are termed as emergency procedures.

Indications

The most common indications for caesarean section are:
- Labour dystocia (i.e. failure to progress)
- Non-reassuring fetal status
- Failed induction of labour (when at least 12–18 hours of oxytocin infusion with adequate contractions and ruptured membranes has failed to effect cervical effacement and dilation)

General risks	Specific risks	Long-term risks
Pain Bleeding, requirement for blood transfusion Infection: wound, urinary, deep Thromboembolism	Injury to bladder, bowel, urinary tract Fetal laceration (1% of cases) Hysterectomy for haemorrhage control	↑ risk of placenta praevia ↑ risk of morbidly adherent placenta (placenta accreta) Scar rupture in subsequent labour (1 in 200 cases) with risks of: • Hysterectomy (10%) • Hypoxic ischaemic encephalopathy (10–50%) • Fetal mortality (10%) • Surgical risks of repeat caesarean

Table 7.7 Caesarean section: risks

- Previous caesarean section (in which case the procedure is termed as an elective repeat caesarean section)
- Medical indication (e.g. placenta praevia or breech presentation)

Primary caesarean sections at maternal request make up a small proportion of all caesareans carried out in the UK.

Risks

The risks of caesarean section are listed in **Table 7.7**. Compared with the risk of maternal mortality in cases of vaginal delivery, the risk in elective caesarean sections is three to five times higher. The risk is higher still in emergency procedures. However, these risks are low in absolute terms. In high-income countries, the incidence of maternal death is about 13 in 100,000 after a caesarean birth, compared with 4 in 100,000 after a vaginal birth. Overall, caesarean section is very safe, and the risk to the individual woman is low, particularly if she is healthy and it is an elective procedure.

Complications arising during labour and delivery

chapter 8

Complications of childbirth are often unanticipated, e.g. prolapse of the umbilical cord. However, the interventions used to manage such complications can be technically challenging and time critical (e.g. caesarean section for cord prolapse).

Dealing with complications and unanticipated events is fundamental to obstetrics. Prediction of risk is difficult, and most obstetric complications that are poorly predicted occur intrapartum.

Complications are divided into two groups:
- Abnormal fetal condition, i.e. fetal compromise, as indicated by pathological changes in cardiotocographic patterns during labour
- Abnormal labour, requiring management that differs from that for an uncomplicated vaginal birth, e.g. augmentation of labour in a case of prolonged labour (also called labour dystocia or failure to progress)

In most instances, abnormal findings on cardiotocography (CTG) do not indicate significant fetal compromise. With appropriate management, many 'abnormal' labours end with an uncomplicated vaginal birth. Conversely, some events and CTG patterns require urgent action in the interests of both fetal and maternal health.

Guiding principle

Any difficult or emergency birth is a frightening experience. Stay calm and in control, and explain briefly to the woman what is happening and that many people will be involved in her care. When possible, obtain written or verbal consent for any intervention.

8.1 Clinical scenario

Unplanned breech birth

Presentation

A woman presents to the birthing suite at 6 am, complaining of labour pains at 39 weeks' gestation. She reports no formal antenatal care to date, although she has had first trimester and 20-week scans through her general practitioner; she says that the results were normal. Past obstetric history is significant for two term caesarean sections. There is no other surgical, medical or psychiatric history. There are no allergies to any medications. The contractions started 2 hours ago, and her membranes ruptured spontaneously in the car on the way to the hospital. She requests an urgent caesarean section.

Examination

Abdominal palpation is poorly tolerated. However, a firm round pole is felt in the upper abdomen. Vaginal examination reveals a 6-cm dilated cervix with a footling breech presentation and an obstetrically narrow pelvis. The consultant obstetrician, anaesthetist and operating theatre staff are urgently alerted. However, progress continues to be rapid and the woman complains of bowel pressure. Repeat examination shows the cervix to be fully dilated with the breech at the ischial spines and one foot at the vaginal introitus (opening).

Management

It is no longer safe to transfer from the birthing suite, because of the real risk of birth in transit and the inability to perform the manoeuvres needed to complete the birth in this setting. Therefore, the woman is placed in the lithotomy position; the vagina anaesthetised with pudendal and perineal infiltration; the maternal bladder emptied by catheter; and the paediatrician and resuscitaire requested in preparation for vaginal delivery.

The woman is encouraged to push with her contractions, and an episiotomy is made as the breech stretches the introitus. Delivery of the breech is completed with Pinard's manoeuvre for the non-footing leg, and the baby allowed to be delivered, with maternal effort, to the armpits. The fetal arms are released with Lovset's manoeuvre. The Mauriceau–Smellie–Veit manoeuvre fails to deliver the fetal head, because of the pelvic dimensions. Therefore, delivery is completed with the help of forceps and the neonate handed to the paediatrician. The remainder of the unplanned birth is uncomplicated. The woman is debriefed.

8.2 Vaginal breech birth

Vaginal delivery of a baby in the breech position is uncommon for several reasons. First, only about 5% of term babies are breech. Second, of the women who do not have a successful external cephalic version (see page 122), most have a caesarean section (as either their choice or the only option available).

Risks Vaginal breech birth is not commonly planned, because of its decreasing familiarity and the results of large trials. Having said this, it remains a reasonable option for clinically suitable women in units who regularly perform planned vaginal breech births, e.g. if the woman is multiparous, has had a healthy pregnancy with normally grown fetus and onset of labour is spontaneous. The risk of complications during elective vaginal breech birth is reduced by ensuring that it is offered to women who are appropriate candidates.

Vaginal breech birth is contraindicated and caesarean section is recommended if:
- The fetus is very large (>4 kg) or very small (<2.5 kg)
- The fetus is known to have pre-existing compromise (e.g. abnormal results from Doppler studies or oligohydramnios)
- There is another indication for caesarean section (e.g. previous caesarean section)
- The breech is anything other than flexed or frank or the facilities for safe vaginal breech birth are unavailable (chapter 5)

Cord prolapse The risk of cord prolapse is highest with the footing breech presentation, because the small diameter of the fetal leg leaves space in the dilated cervix for entry of the cord. Cord prolapse occurs in one in five footing breech deliveries.

Therefore, caesarean section is required. If cord prolapse occurs during birth, it is managed as for cases of cord prolapse in cephalic presentations (see page 204).

Head entrapment This complication is most likely in cases of breech delivery of a preterm baby. This is because the head of a preterm fetus has the largest diameter of any part of its body, and the fetal buttocks is occasionally delivered before the cervix is sufficiently dilated to allow passage of the head.

- If the cervix is incompletely dilated, Duhrssen's incisions are made in the cervix at the 2, 6 and 10 o'clock positions to increase space for the fetal head
- If the cervix is fully dilated, head flexion is aided by any combination of suprapubic pressure, Mariceau–Smellie–Veit manoeuvre and forceps to deliver the after-coming head for added leverage

Fetal injury The most common injury associated with vaginal breech birth is limb fracture. However, bones heal with excellent results in neonates. Less common are nerve palsies, spinal injury from extreme flexion or extension, and intracranial haemorrhage. Paediatric review is recommended for all vaginally delivered breech babies.

Diagnostic approach

Ultrasound is used to determine the position of the fetal legs (flexed, frank or footling) and the attitude of the fetal head. Footling breech and extended neck are contraindications to vaginal breech birth, because of the high risk of cord prolapse, cervical spine injury and head entrapment.

Management

Continuous CTG is used to monitor fetal condition. A senior colleague is informed of the situation. If labour is progressing slowly, no attempt is made to use oxytocin to augment it and caesarean section is performed as it is safer for the baby. If the cardiotocograph is indicative of fetal compromise, urgent caesarean section is carried out for the same reason.

When the second stage of labour begins, the woman's bladder is emptied, which can be aided by a catheter if necessary, and the paediatric team requested. The woman is encouraged to push with contractions and any spontaneous urges. The perineum is infiltrated with local anaesthetic in preparation for episiotomy. If access is needed, an episiotomy is made when the buttocks crown. At this point, the urge to intervene must be resisted ('hands off the breech'), because this causes extension of the fetal arm and head, which makes delivery more challenging. The baby must never be pulled. **Figure 8.1** shows the manoeuvres used in a vaginal breech delivery.

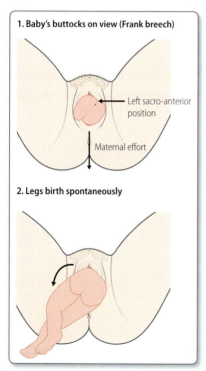

Figure 8.1 Vaginal breech birth: delivery technique. Pinard's manoeuvre can also be performed in stage 2 by flexing each knee and flexing the leg laterally, causing it to birth. *Continues on pages 202–203.*

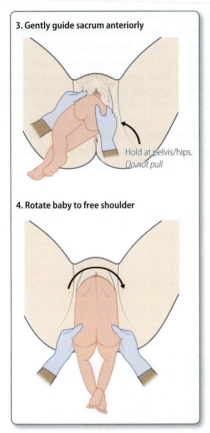

Figure 8.1 Continued.

Management of the third stage proceeds as for an uncomplicated vaginal delivery.

Postpartum care The baby is assessed by a paediatrician at birth. A clinical hip examination is carried out on the postnatal ward. A hip US study is requested for the baby at 6 weeks of age, because breech babies are at increased risk of developmental dysplasia of the hip.

Vaginal breech birth 203

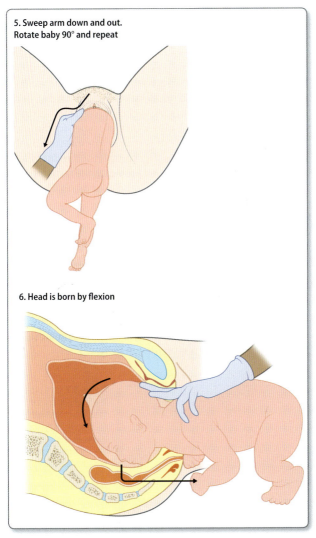

Figure 8.1 *Continued.*

8.3 Cord prolapse

In cord prolapse, the umbilical cord descends with or past a presenting part of the fetus (**Figure 8.2**). In occult cord prolapse, the cord descends alongside the presenting part. Cord prolapse may be detected indirectly, when cardiotocographic abnormalities appear (e.g. deep variable deceleration or bradycardia), or directly, when the cord is felt in the vagina or seen at the introitus.

The umbilical cord is the only source of oxygen for the fetus. In cases of prolapse, the cord is usually compressed by the presenting parts of the fetus. The compression reduces fetal oxygen supply, and if not relieved promptly, the resulting fetal hypoxia can lead to permanent disability or death. Therefore, cord prolapse is a true obstetric emergency.

Management

Management of cord prolapse has two goals: to relieve cord compression and thus increase fetal oxygenation, and to carry out timely delivery by caesarean section (unless the cervix is fully dilated or the fetus previable).

The procedure in cases of cord prolapse is as follows:
- If there has been no monitoring of fetal heart rate (especially if the woman has arrived at hospital with cord prolapse), US is used to check for fetal cardiac activity

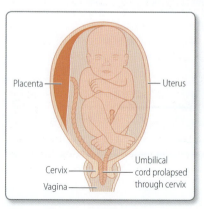

Figure 8.2 Cord prolapse. The fetus is in complete breech presentation, the placenta is on the lateral uterine wall, and the umbilical cord has prolapsed through the cervix into the vagina.

- Help is summoned by pressing the emergency buzzer
- The woman is asked to roll on to all fours and elevate her buttocks in the air. Any exposed cord is placed in the vagina to minimise the risk of vasospasm in response to cold and pressure as this decreases blood flow to the fetus; it is not handled further. A gloved hand is placed in the vagina and used to push up the presenting part of the fetus, thereby raising it above the cervix to help relieve cord compression (if the woman has an indwelling catheter, another option is to fill the bladder with 500 cm^3 of warm saline and then clamp the catheter; the full bladder elevates the fetus)
- The woman is transported to the operating theatre in this position for an urgent caesarean section
- Fetal cardiac activity is checked again before the first incision. The gloved hand is not removed from the vagina until the woman is under general anaesthesia and the operating surgeon asks for the hand to be removed

Prognosis

If cord prolapse occurs in hospital, the fetus has previously been well, and the appropriate measures are taken, neonatal outcome is good. However, the experience is traumatic for the mother.

> **Clinical insight**
>
> To preserve dignity a sheet is used to cover the woman's buttocks while she is transported to the operating theatre for caesarean section, because she must remain on all fours with a clinician keeping a gloved vaginal hand to avoid umbilical cord compression.

8.4 Shoulder dystocia

Shoulder dystocia occurs during vaginal birth when the anterior fetal shoulder impacts against the maternal pubic symphysis (**Figure 8.3**). This creates a mechanical obstruction to delivery of the rest of the body that cannot be overcome by maternal effort. The consequences are cord compression and inexorable fetal hypoxia, acidosis and demise if the shoulder dystocia is not relieved. The incidence is about 1% of all births.

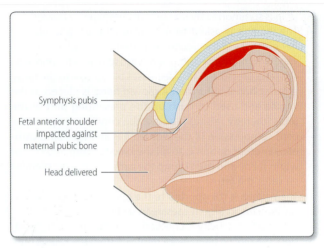

Figure 8.3 Shoulder dystocia.

Aetiology
In cases of prior history of shoulder dystocia, the risk of recurrence is 10%. Other risk factors for shoulder dystocia (**Table 8.1**) are all poorly predictive. Half of all cases occur in women with no risk factors.

Diagnostic approach
Shoulder dystocia is diagnosed when the head has been delivered but retracts back on to the perineum ('turtles') or routine traction fails to deliver the shoulders.

Management
Management of shoulder dystocia is one of the most challenging experiences for an obstetrician. All obstetric first-line caregivers must know the steps of management as it is unpredictable and urgent. However, it is essential to remain calm and reassuring, because the woman will feel powerless and frightened.

The obstructed shoulder is disimpacted by carrying out a series of manoeuvres that increase the pelvic diameters or rotate the shoulder into the oblique plane.

Category	Factors
Maternal	Obesity (surrogate marker for fetal macrosomia and diabetes) Diabetes (altered fetal anthropometry, with wider shoulders) Contracted pelvis due to trauma, stature or rickets (rare) History of shoulder dystocia (personal phenotype of risk)
Fetal	Macrosomia Post-term gestation
Labour	Induction of labour Augmentation of labour, especially when at advanced cervical dilation Slow progress Prolonged second stage Instrumental delivery

Table 8.1 Shoulder dystocia: risk factors

'**HELPERR**' is a useful mnemonic for management of shoulder dystopia.

> **Clinical insight**
>
> A clear request is made for the paediatrician and resuscitaire. They are often forgotten in the urgency of attempts to deliver the baby.

- **H**: call for Help.
- **E**: move the woman to the Edge of the bed. This gives access for internal manoeuvres. Consider Epsiotomy for access; however, in practice, if not already done, this is technically challenging with the fetal cheeks on the maternal perineum. Anticipate the possibility of severe perineal trauma, postpartum haemorrhage (PPH) or fetal trauma
- **L**: elevate the Legs with the McRoberts manoeuvre ('knees to nipples' hyperflexion of the hips). This flattens the lumbar lordosis and increases pelvic diameters. It will relieve 50–90% of shoulder dystocias
- **P**: apply suprapubic Pressure from the direction of the fetal back to dislodge the obstructed shoulder into the oblique plane
- **E**: Enter the vagina and perform internal manoeuvres to rotate the obstructed shoulder into the oblique plane. These include Woods' screw, reverse Woods' screw (rotating the entire baby either forwards or backwards into the oblique

plane to free the shoulder under the symphysis by means of digital pressure on the back and shoulders, like turning a tap with a two-handed grip), delivery of the posterior arm, and axillary sling traction and rotation
- **R**: Roll over and repeat the same manoeuvres with the woman on all fours, because this also increases pelvic diameters
- **R**: Repeat all manoeuvres. Consider the final options for vaginal delivery, which are deliberate clavicular fracture, maternal symphysiotomy (division of the pubic symphysis). The final option for attempted live fetal salvage is to perform Zavenelli's manoeuvre (by which the delivered fetal head is pushed back into the vagina) followed by caesarean section. Zavenelli's manoeuvre is associated with high morbidity for mother and baby, and most fetuses have anoxic brain injuries if born alive by this method.

8.5 Inverted uterus

Uterine inversion is the invagination and prolapse of the uterine fundus through the cervix (**Figure 8.4**). In extreme cases, the uterus is entirely inverted and visible at the vaginal introitus.

Rapid diagnosis and management of uterine inversion is paramount, because it is not a benign occurrence: it leads to maternal death via neurogenic and haemorrhagic shock.

Aetiology

Risk factors for uterine inversion relate to poor detachment of the placenta, traction on a non-separated placenta or mechanical predisposition to inversion. They are:
- Morbidly adherent placenta (accreta)
- Traction before placental separation
- Fundal placenta
- Short umbilical cord
- Previous uterine inversion

Uterine inversion is rare, occurring in about 1 in 2000 births. Therefore, most cases are unexpected and risk factor assessment is unhelpful.

Inverted uterus 209

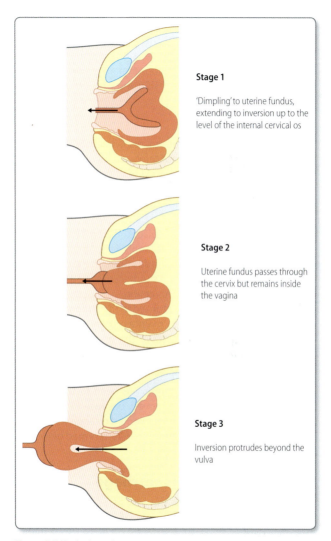

Stage 1

'Dimpling' to uterine fundus, extending to inversion up to the level of the internal cervical os

Stage 2

Uterine fundus passes through the cervix but remains inside the vagina

Stage 3

Inversion protrudes beyond the vulva

Figure 8.4 Uterine inversion.

Diagnostic approach

The diagnosis is obvious if the fundus appears at the introitus with cord traction. Other signs include a dimpled or impalpable uterine fundus abdominally, especially in the presence of maternal hypotension from neurogenic shock and PPH.

Management

It is directed at replacing the uterus, resolving shock, resuscitating and delivering the placenta safely.

All attempts to deliver with cord traction are stopped. The emergency buzzer is pressed to summon help. The woman is informed about what is happening, what is being done and why this is necessary.

A gentle attempt is made to replace the uterus (called reduction) by using a gloved hand to apply firm, steady pressure upwards, thereby pushing the fundus through the cervix. Care is taken not to apply force in one site, because the uterus is soft and would be perforated by this action.

Once the uterus has been returned to the abdominal cavity, oxytocin infusion is started to maintain uterine tone. Urgent manual removal of the placenta in the operating theatre is arranged so there is access to adequate general anaesthesia and skilled help to complete the procedure.

Postpartum care Once the uterus has been restored to the abdomen and the placenta removed, because PPH is anticipated, both this and reinversion prevented by aggressive treatment with oxytocic agents. The woman is informed of the risk of recurrence in subsequent births.

8.6 Postpartum haemorrhage

Postpartum haemorrhage is the loss of ≥500 mL from the genital tract after vaginal delivery or the loss of ≥750 mL at caesarean section. It is a cause of significant maternal morbidity and a leading direct cause of maternal mortality. About 15% of all births are affected.

Postpartum haemorrhage can be both massive and rapid, because of the large blood supply to the uterus at term. Prompt recognition, resuscitation and treatment to stop the bleeding are essential.

Classification

Postpartum haemorrhage is classified by its timing.

> **Clinical insight**
>
> Be suspicious of the diagnosis of 'secondary PPH' occurring >4–6 weeks after the birth. In most cases, it is a period.

- Primary PPH occurs within 24 hours of birth
- Secondary PPH occurs from 24 hours to 6 weeks after childbirth. It is caused by subinvolution (failure of the uterus to return to its non-gravid state) due to infection or the presence of retained placental tissue

Postpartum haemorrhage is also classified by blood loss. This is because the volume of blood lost is a more important factor than timing when determining immediate management and the risk of complications.

- **Minor PPH**: 500–1000 mL
- **Major PPH**: 1000–2000 mL
- **Severe PPH**: 2000–2500 mL
- **'Mega' PPH**: >2500 mL

Primary postpartum haemorrhage

Primary PPH occurs in the first 24 hours after birth. Of its many causes (**Table 8.2**), loss of uterine tone accounts for 90% of cases. Fetal macrosomia obesity and advanced maternal age are associated with increased risk of primary PPH.

Although most PPHs are minor and have little sequelae, this is established in retrospect. All PPHs are obstetric emergencies and require urgent assessment and management becuase of the threat to the mother's wellbeing from rapid blood loss.

Diagnosis

Primary PPH is usually self-evident. It is characterised by active and ongoing vaginal bleeding after birth. This is usually accompanied by signs and symptoms of maternal tachycardia, hypotension and shock.

Cause	Risk factors
Tone (loss of uterine)	Large uterus: grand multiparity, polyhydramnios, multiple gestation, macrosomia, fibroids Poorly contractile uterus: precipitate labour, long labour, prolonged second stage, augmentation of labour, maternal neuromuscular disease, chorioamnionitis, physiological third stage, placenta praevia, nulliparity, idiopathic, previous PPH Traumatised uterus: inversion, rupture
Tissue	Retained placenta or membranes, succenturiate lobe, bipartite placenta and other variations in placental shape
Trauma	Cervical laceration, lower genital tract trauma (including vaginal and perineal laceration), episiotomy, instrumental vaginal delivery
Thrombin (low)	Consumptive coagulopathy (inability to clot due to use of body's store of available coagulation factors) in established PPH, placental abruption and pre-eclampsia, sepsis, amniotic fluid embolism, congenital coagulopathy (e.g. von Willebrand's disease)
PPH, postpartum haemorrhage.	

Table 8.2 Primary postpartum haemorrhage: causes

Clinical insight

Remember that estimates of blood loss are unreliable (as blood soaks into bedding and pads and is mopped away, as well as being mixed with maternal bodily fluids and liquor) and bleeding is occasionally hidden (e.g. behind a partially separated placenta in the uterus). Until proven otherwise, signs of shock are always treated as significant bleeding, regardless of documented blood loss.

Management

The aims of management are to:
- Stop the bleeding
- Identify the cause
- Resuscitate the mother
- Prevent complications

Initial management The aim of initial management is to stop the bleeding, stabilise the mother and streamline rapid transit to theatre if the bleeding continues. Proceed as described below:

Call for help The emergency buzzer is pressed to summon help. An assistant notes when the woman gave birth, whether the placenta has been delivered, the estimated blood loss, the resuscitation and oxytocic agent given, and the vital signs (if known).

Stop the bleeding Multiple oxytocic agents (**Table 8.3**) are given in order of suitability, availability and familiarity. Uterine contraction is stimulated manually by rubbing the uterine fundus to stimulate a tonic contraction to facilitate the expulsion of clots and encourage uterine tone.

> **Guiding principle**
>
> A scribe is a clinician who takes on the sole duty of documenting events and treatments for later record and to guide the treatment team in what has already been attempted and when it was done. This is invaluable in a chaotic emergency. They are useful as a prompter and timekeeper, asking questions such as 'Have we given rectal misoprostol?'

Drug	Mechanism of action	Risks and precautions
Synthetic oxytocin (Syntocinon)	Stimulates uterine contractions	Hypotension and arrhythmia when given rapidly intravenously Antidiuresis
Ergometrine	Stimulates tonic and lasting uterine contractions	Contraindicated in hypertension, exacerbates vasospasm Vomiting common – give with antiemetic
Misoprostol	Stimulates uterine contractions, long-lasting	Slow onset – give early Febrile response, which may be mistaken for sepsis
Carboprost (Hemabate, prostaglandin F2α)	Potent stimulator of uterine contractions	Vomiting (common), hypertension, bronchospasm, flushing, fever
Tranexamic acid	Antifibrinolytic, stabilises clot	Nausea, headache, diarrhoea, theoretical prothrombotic risk

Table 8.3 Postpartum haemorrhage: medications

An indwelling catheter is placed. Adding a urinometer allows subsequent assessment of hourly urine output.

Bleeding perineal tears are sutured promptly or have pressure applied to them. The placenta is examined. If it is incomplete, urgent manual removal in theatre of the retained parts is arranged.

Resuscitate and monitor A 'DRABC' approach is followed (see page 134). Two 16-gauge IV cannulae are placed in large veins, and the blood specimens obtained are sent for cross-matching, full blood examination and coagulation profile. Between 1 and 2 L of warmed saline is given by rapid infusion; more can be given, as needed. Observations of heart rate, respiratory rate, saturations and blood pressure are recorded every 15 minutes. Hourly urine output is also checked and documented. Use of a pulse oximeter provides continuous information on heart rate, which is useful for identifying evolving tachycardia.

Reduce complications A warmed blanket is placed around the woman to avoid worsening of the coagulopathy. Supine hypotension is avoided by placing a wedge under her right hip; this displaces the uterus to relieve pressure on the great vessels. When haemostasis has been achieved, thromboembolism is prevented by mechanical compression and pharmacological prophylaxis. In cases of severe perineal trauma or injury to the uterine lining, IV broad-spectrum antibiotics are given to reduce the risk of endometritis and wound breakdown.

Document When the bleeding has settled to normal postpartum loss, the loss is estimated by weighing all pads, towels and sheets and the total recorded. Intravenous fluid replacement is used to balance this deficit. After 2–3 L of fluid has been given, blood products are generally required, because excessive infusion of saline worsens acidosis, dilutes coagulation factors and disrupts coagulation. In life-threatening cases, emergency blood is requested; all midwifery units and hospitals maintain O-negative, Kell-negative blood for the treatment of haemorrhage.

Postpartum haemorrhage 215

In-theatre care If bleeding from the uterus continues, the woman is taken quickly to the operating theatre. On the way, torrential bleeding is stopped temporarily by bimanual uterine compression (**Figure 8.5**); this is lifesaving. **Table 8.4** shows the options when the bleeding is from a source other than the uterus.

> **Clinical insight**
>
> Tachycardia is the first sign of blood loss. In healthy women, it is often the only sign of haemorrhage until advanced shock ensues. This is indicated by hypotension, tachypnoea, confusion and air hunger experienced as subjective shortness of breath.

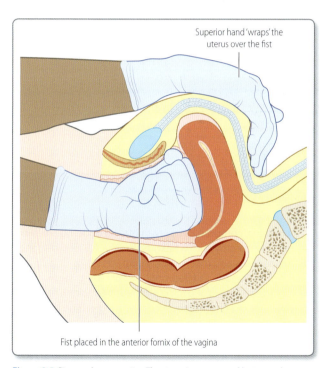

Figure 8.5 Bimanual compression. The uterus is compressed between the upper hand on the abdomen, pushing down on the fundus, and the lower hand in the vagina.

Source of bleeding	Management options
Cervix	Examine cervix for lacerations Suture bleeding tears
Lower genital tract	Suture bleeding tears
No source identified	Diagnose coagulopathy; inform anaesthetist; give tranexamic acid, platelets and coagulation factors; pack or tamponade uterus

Table 8.4 Postpartum haemorrhage: management for non-uterine sources of bleeding

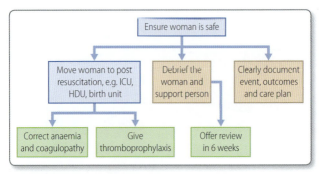

Figure 8.6 Follow-up care for postpartum haemorrhage.

If bimanual compression gains control of ongoing bleeding, tamponade therapy with a Bakri balloon (a balloon designed to fill the uterus and mechanically compress bleeding points) is used. The balloon is filled until the bleeding stops or the maximum capacity of 500 mL is reached. It remains in utero for no longer than 24 hours, because beyond this time the risk of uterine necrosis and infection is unacceptably high.

If other measures have failed or the woman is moribund, surgical control is required. This is achieved by laparotomy followed by placement of B-Lynch uterine compression sutures, uterine artery ligation and hysterectomy (for definitive resolution).

Follow-up care Major PPH events require transfer to a monitored setting so that recognition of complications and appropriate transfusion is prompt (**Figure 8.6**). The mother receives early postpartum care. This includes assistance with breastfeeding. If she is too unwell to feed the baby, she is helped to express breast milk. Breastfeeding and breast milk expression are psychologically beneficial and promote physiological changes that promote uterine contraction.

Postnatal care

chapter 9

The postpartum period extends for 6 weeks from delivery. It requires a multidisciplinary approach to care. An obstetrics and gynaecology specialist, a paediatrician, a general practitioner, a midwife and a maternal and child health nurse work together to ensure optimal health of the mother and baby and early recognition of any complications.

9.1 Clinical scenario
Breastfeeding difficulties
Presentation
A 26-year-old teacher presents 2 weeks after birth with a 4-day history of a painful left breast, fever, lethargy and myalgia. She normally breastfeeds her baby every 3 hours, but for the last 2 days, she has been breastfeeding him every 4–5 hours because of the tenderness in her breast. The tenderness is localised to the left breast only and is getting progressively worse.

On further questioning, she mentions that she has been unhappy and teary, because she feels overwhelmed by life as a new mother. She no longer derives pleasure from activities she enjoyed previously. These feelings began last week.

Breast examination reveals that, compared with the right breast, the left breast is slightly swollen and erythematous. It is tender on palpation. No masses or abnormal nipple discharge or damage is detected. Body temperature is 38.5°C. Other vital signs are within their normal ranges. Examination of the newborn shows appropriate growth and hydration.

Diagnostic approach
Unilateral mastalgia in a breastfeeding woman with flu-like symptoms is the classic presentation of mastitis (inflammation of breast tissue due to accumulation of breast milk and subsequent infection). In this case, the woman's normal body temperature and vital signs rule out an underlying sepsis.

She is asked to describe how she feeds the baby, because incorrect technique can cause trauma to the nipple. This results in reluctance to use the affected breast for feeding, and mastitis ensues.

Her deflated emotional state, tendency to cry and anhedonia are attributed to the onset of baby blues, the low mood experienced by some mothers in the postpartum period. She is asked about:
- Any changes in appetite, weight or sleeping pattern that suggest postnatal depression
- Medications that interfere with mood
- Support from family, friends or the community

The baby's good health on examination is an excellent sign. However, the reduction in breastfeeding frequency due to the breast tenderness and the mother's depressed mood could lead to failure to gain weight and dehydration.

Further investigations

No investigations are required, because the clinical presentation is typical of mastitis. However, tests are carried out to exclude conditions that mimic mastitis.
- The results of full blood examination and measurement of inflammatory markers rule out an inflammatory condition
- A US scan of the breast shows normal breast tissue parenchyma with no abscesses or tumours, ruling out an abscess or, very rarely, inflammatory breast cancer

A depression screen is administered to establish whether a diagnosis of depressive disorder would be appropriate. The results show anhedonia, low mood and poor concentration. A Mini-Mental State Examination gives a score of 29 out of 30, indicating normal cognition. Thyroid function test results are within the normal ranges. These findings, along with the short duration and mild nature of the symptoms, exclude depression, psychosis and thyroiditis and are consistent with baby blues.

Management

The woman is started on a course of oral antibiotics to treat the mild infection underlying the mastitis. She is also advised to continue

> **Clinical insight**
>
> Stasis of breast milk results in growth of infectious organisms. Therefore, promotion of fluid motion is a key aim of treatment for mastitis.

breastfeeding or expressing, because emptying the breast of accumulated milk relieves the tenderness and minimises further bacterial growth. To treat the baby blues, her partner is encouraged to help her resume the activities she used to enjoy before giving birth. Five days later, her breast symptoms have disappeared and her mental state has returned to normal.

9.2 Breastfeeding

Breastfeeding difficulties should be recognised and addressed, because they are detrimental to mother–baby bonding and growth of the newborn (**Table 9.1**). Breastfeeding has benefits for both baby and mother, however approximately 5% of women have inadequate milk supply and supplemental formula milk is required. In a First World country with clean water supplies, many women will choose formula milk for social, employment and other feeding difficulty reasons.

Benefits

Exclusive breastfeeding is recommended for the baby's first 4–6 months, because the components of breast milk are more nutritious, better absorbed by the baby's gastrointestinal system, and provide immunological value. The benefits for both the mother and baby are outlined in **Table 9.2**.

> **Clinical insight**
>
> The World Health Organization, in collaboration with the United Nations Children's Fund, has established the Baby-friendly Hospital Initiative, a 10-step programme to encourage midwifery units, hospitals and other organisations providing maternity care to adopt changes that promote and support breastfeeding.

Breastfeeding difficulty	Manifestation	Management
Inadequate milk supply	Frequent short feeding times Maternal frustration or depression Baby fails to thrive, and demonstrates signs of hunger with excessive crying and frequent feeding cues (rooting, lip-smacking and sucking) Few wet nappies in a 24-hour period >10% birthweight loss and slow weight gain	Lactation consultant review Advise mother on good nutrition Regular breastfeeding or breast milk expression (expressed milk is given by bottle until the supply is adequate) Formula supplementation Pharmacological galactagogue (dopamine agonist such as domperidone)
Overfeeding	Baby vomits or chokes on rapid let down of milk Frothy stools	Change feeding routine Expressing let down to avoid choking Correct feeding technique Educate on signs of a completely fed baby
Cracked nipples	Stinging and burning nipples, especially during feeding Bleeding from skin around the nipples and red excoriated areolae	Encourage proper attachment and latching on Recommend feeding baby with expressed milk by bottle while nipples heal

Table 9.1 Breastfeeding difficulties and their management

Contraindications

Breastfeeding is largely safe for the mother and baby. However, it is contraindicated in the following cases:
- Active maternal HIV or tuberculosis infection
- Maternal treatment for malignant neoplasm
- Misuse of alcohol or other substances
- Galactosaemia in the infant

Mother	Baby
• Better mother–baby psychological bonding, which hastens recovery after birth • Protection against mild mood changes, including baby blues • Decreased risk of bleeding, including postpartum haemorrhage, because oxytocin released during breastfeeding promotes shrinkage of the uterus to its pre-pregnancy size • Moderate contraceptive effect, because prolactin secreted during breastfeeding causes amenorrhoea • Reduced risk of epithelial ovarian cancer, due to delayed ovulation • Reduced risk of premenopausal breast cancer, because oestrogen levels are lower • Financial benefits and convenience: breast milk is free and available at any time, without the need for special facilities or equipment (other than a breast pump, if required)	• Protection against middle ear and other upper respiratory tract infections • Fewer gastrointestinal tract infections (e.g. gastroenteritis) • Lower likelihood of developing atopic conditions (e.g. asthma and eczema) and allergies • Resistance to childhood obesity and juvenile diabetes • Improved psychological and social development, because breastfeeding fosters emotional closeness

Table 9.2 Benefits of breastfeeding for the mother and baby

9.3 Maternal mental health

Significant morbidity and mortality is associated with mental illness during and after pregnancy. After giving birth, mothers face challenges from three groups of factors. These have the potential to negatively affect her mental state.

- **Biological:** physical changes due to rapid hormonal fluctuations during labour and lactation
- **Emotional:** coping with exhaustion and pain; difficulty in bonding with or caring for the baby; pressure to recover former body shape; anxiety about resuming the sexual

relationship with the partner; and changing relationships with the partner, family members and friends
- **Social:** financial, family support and housing considerations, and worries about prospects for progression in employment or education

> ### Guiding principle
> A mother's mental well-being has a significant influence on her baby's mental health and development. Early recognition and treatment of maternal postnatal mental illness helps protect the child from long-term emotional, behavioural and intellectual problems.

Baby (postpartum) blues

Baby blues is the name for the low mood caused by the hormonal fluctuations of labour, the exhausting process of giving birth and the challenges of caring for a newborn. It is experienced by up to 60–80% of new mothers. Women from lower socioeconomic backgrounds are particularly vulnerable.

Clinical features
The mother experiences any combination of lethargy, tearfulness, sleep disruption, loss of concentration, anxiety and irritability. These symptoms start within 4–5 days of delivery.

Management
Baby blues resolves spontaneously within a few days of onset. Management includes reassurance to the mother, supporting the mother in caring for the baby, and allowing as much rest as possible. Given the mild and transient nature of the symptoms, pharmacological therapy is unnecessary and therefore not recommended.

Perinatal depression

Perinatal depression is characterised by depressive symptoms associated with the peripartum period. It is present with significant mood and behavioural changes that may or may not be against a background of known psychiatric illness.

Clinical features
Symptoms of postnatal depression include anhedonia, depressed mood, weight loss, sleep interruption, psychomotor retardation

(slowness of thoughts and physical activity), fatigue, loss of concentration and, in extreme cases, suicidal ideation.

Management

It starts with supportive measures: discussing feelings with family, friends and support groups, and cognitive behavioural therapy sessions. If this initial strategy is ineffective, antidepressants are added in consultation with a psychiatrist. Separation from the baby is avoided, because it exacerbates the condition.

Severe cases that do not respond to outpatient therapy, or where there is a risk of self-harm or harm to the baby, require admission to a mother–baby unit urgently for inpatient specialist psychiatric treatment.

Postpartum psychosis

Postpartum psychosis is an uncommon but severe condition. It affects women with a history of bipolar disorder or postpartum psychosis after a previous birth.

Clinical features

The symptoms are a mix of depression and mania. Early symptoms are non-specific and include disturbed sleep, poor concentration and irritability. After a few weeks, the symptoms include pressured speech, hallucinations and delusions, accompanied by either elevated mood and high energy or depressed mood and anhedonia. At this stage, the mother may have suicidal and homicidal ideas. Therefore, prompt recognition and treatment are essential.

Management

Treatment requires admission to hospital, urgent psychiatric evaluation, administration of antipsychotic medication and continuous observation. Separation from the baby is avoided if possible, but is warranted in severe cases.

If symptoms fail to improve, management includes electroconvulsive therapy. The aggressiveness of treatment reflects the high incidence of infanticide (up to 4%) and suicide associated with this condition.

All women who have had an episode of postpartum psychosis are at increased risk of subsequent bipolar disorder, and postpartum psychosis in future pregnancies.

9.4 Postpartum pyrexia and sepsis

Postpartum pyrexia is characterised by a maternal body temperature of ≥38°C lasting at least 24 hours within the first 10 days of delivery. Its multiple causes are divided into four groups. From most to least common causes, these are as follows:
- **Breast disorders:** mastitis and breast abscess
- **Urogenital tract infections:** endometritis and urinary tract infection or pyelonephritis
- **Other infections:** gastroenteritis, pneumonia, epidural abscess and surgical site infections
- **Inflammation:** deep vein thrombosis and pulmonary embolism

> **Guiding principle**
>
> The cause of fever requires urgent identification. Any delay could lead to sepsis, which is life-threatening (see page 232).

All cases of postpartum pyrexia require full blood examination and measurement of inflammatory markers (especially C-reactive protein). Blood cultures are taken, along with vaginal and wound (perineal or caesarean) swabs and urine culture. Other investigations depend on the signs, symptoms and systems involved in the febrile presentation. Risk factors for postpartum pyrexia are listed in **Table 9.3**.

Mastitis

Mastitis is inflammation of the breast parenchyma due to obstruction of milk ducts and consequent milk stasis. Most cases of mastitis are caused by bacteria (usually *Staphylococcus aureus*), which colonise the milk that accumulates in the breast.

Clinical features

Most women report classic flu-like symptoms and breast pain. Unilateral breast engorgement, tenderness and erythema

Category	Risk factors
Lifestyle	Obesity Smoking Substance abuse Poor hygiene or sanitation Immobility
Obstetric	Caesarean section Indwelling urinary catheter or IV cannula Spinal or epidural anaesthesia Intrapartum pyrexia Chorioamnionitis Prolonged rupture of membranes, prolonged labour Retained products of conception
Other medical conditions	Diabetes Immunosuppression

Table 9.3 Postpartum pyrexia: risk factors

are present. They are associated with ipsilateral tender or enlarged axillary lymph nodes.

Investigations
No investigations are required, because this is a clinical diagnosis. However, normal findings on a full blood examination and C-reactive protein measurement may help exclude severe sepsis. Persistence of symptoms for >7 days prompts investigation with blood tests for markers of inflammation (white cell count, CRP), bacteraemia (blood culture), breast ultrasound (to exclude complicating abscess as nadir for continued symptoms) and breast milk for culture. Areolar fungal swabs should also be performed (as nipple thrush has symptoms which can mislead the diagnosis.

Management
Simple cases of mastitis are treated with a 5- to 7-day course of an oral antibiotic agent, typically flucloxacillin, which is effec-

tive against *S. aureus* (the most common causative organism). Simple analgesia with paracetamol (acetaminophen), which is also an effective antipyretic, relieves the breast tenderness as well as reduces the fever.

Breast abscess

A breast abscess is a localised collection of pus in inflamed breast tissue. It is usually secondary to mastitis.

Clinical features
Breast abscess is characterised by features of mastitis plus a palpable tender and fluctuant discrete breast mass associated with fluctuating fever.

Investigations
A US scan of the breast identifies the abscess and guides aspiration of purulent fluid for culture.

Management
Compared with mastitis, breast abscess requires a longer course (up to 14 days) of oral antibiotics. Simple analgesia, antipyretics, and removal of the pus by abscess drainage are also needed.

Endometritis

Endometritis is an inflammation of the endometrium, most commonly in response to an infection ascending from the lower genital tract.

Clinical features
Uterine tenderness and bleeding characterise endometritis.

Investigations
A high vaginal swab sample is obtained for culture.

Management
Broad-spectrum IV antibiotics covering anaerobic bacteria are used. These include ampicillin, gentamicin and metronidazole.

Urinary tract infection and pyelonephritis

Urinary tract infections and pyelonephritis are inflammation of the lower and upper urinary tract, respectively. They are predominantly caused by *Escherichia coli*.

Clinical features

Dysuria, haematuria, pyuria, nocturia and frequency of urination are features of both conditions. Suprapubic, flank or renal angle tenderness are usually present.

Investigations

Urine culture and sensitivity is the mainstay investigation. They are used to identify the causative organism and determine antibiotic sensitivity, which guides appropriate therapy.

Management

If an indwelling urinary catheter is still in situ, it is removed. Oral antibiotics are given for lower urinary tract infection, and parenteral antibiotics for pyelonephritis. The specific antibiotic agent used depends on the antibiotic sensitivity of the causative organism, but initial empiric therapy is initiated as diagnostic results take 24–48 hours. Ceftriaxone is a common agent.

Gastroenteritis

Gastroenteritis is an infection of the gastrointestinal tract, especially the small and large bowels. It is caused by viruses, bacteria or antibiotic use (due to change in intestinal flora associated with antibiotic use).

Clinical features

Signs of dehydration due to diarrhoea are present. The diarrhoea is associated with abdominal cramps. The faeces are blood-stained in bacterial causes, but the absence of blood is not sufficiently reliable to exclude a bacterial cause. The most serious cause is *Listeria* which causes enteritis in immunosuppressed individuals, such as those who are pregnant or who have recently given birth.

Investigations
Stool culture and sensitivity is required to identify the organisms causing the gastroenteritis.

Management
Usually, rehydration with electrolyte-rich oral preparations is needed to address the fluid loss from diarrhoea. If infection is suspected or confirmed from the stool culture, oral antibiotics covering anaerobes (e.g. metronidazole) are given.

Pneumonia
Pneumonia is inflammation of the lung parenchyma caused by various infective organisms, chemicals and environmental exposure to harmful substances.

Clinical features
Pneumonia is characterised by tachypnoea, coarse crepitations on chest auscultation and reduced oxygen saturation.

Investigations
Sputum analysis and culture is used to identify the causative organism(s). A chest X-ray shows the area of lung affected.

Management
Pneumonia is treated with oral or IV antibiotics, depending on the severity. The severity is gauged using the 'CORB' system. Each letter in the **CORB** acronym refers to a feature of pneumonia and is given a score of 1 point.
- **C:** new Confusion
- **O:** Oxygen saturation less or equal to 90% on room air
- **R:** Respiratory rate more or equal to 30 breaths per minute
- **B:** Blood pressure:
    - Systolic <90 mmHg
    - Diastolic ≤60 mmHg

A CORB score of 2–4 indicates severe pneumonia, which requires IV antibiotic therapy with azithromycin. A score below 2 is mild pneumonia and requires an oral antibiotic agent such as amoxicillin or doxycycline. Young adults may not score highly on such systems until critically unwell. A mother with a new baby should be admitted for parenteral treatment in all but the mildest of cases. Remember influenza is a differential diagnosis and is treated with respiratory isolation and antiviral therapy.

Epidural abscess

An epidural abscess is the result of a suppurative infection of the epidural space after administration of epidural or spinal anaesthesia. Most cases are caused by *S. aureus* and are considered a neurological emergency.

Clinical features

The features of epidural abscess are localised midline back pain over the injection site and focal neurological symptoms, including paraesthesia and radicular pain radiating from the lower back to the lower limbs, most commonly unilaterally. Motor deficit, in the form of reduced power, can also be present, especially if the abscess is pressing on a spinal nerve.

Investigations

An imaging study of the spine is needed: MRI, or if MRI is not available, CT scan with the use of a contrast agent. Images of the collection of pus that forms the abscess, facilitate its drainage.

Management

Fluid aspiration alongside administration of IV antibiotics is the most effective treatment for epidural abscess. A prolonged course is required.

Surgical site infection

Infection of an area where recent surgery has been carried out can cause postnatal pyrexia. The two most common sites in obstetrics are those of episiotomy repair and caesarean section.

Clinical features

The site shows local erythema, tenderness and induration associated with wound dehiscence and pus discharge.

Investigations

Full blood examination is required to look for leucocytosis. A wound swab sample is also obtained and sent for culture.

> **Clinical insight**
>
> If the causes of postpartum pyrexia described in this section have been excluded, causes of fever unrelated to pregnancy and delivery are considered. A thorough sexual, travel, medication, family and social history provides useful information. The woman is asked specifically about contact with people who have recently been or are unwell.

Management

Drainage (clearing the wound of pus) and debridement (surgical removal of necrotised tissue) are carried out, if the woman is septic, the collection is not draining spontaneously or conservative management fails. Dressings are applied. Surgical closure of the wound is deferred to allow healing via secondary intention (natural closure after surgery) while the patient is on a course of oral or IV antibiotics.

Maternal sepsis

If maternal infection is not adequately managed, life-threatening organ dysfunction may develop—this is termed as maternal sepsis. While rare in developed countries due to improved hygiene standards and effective treatment of maternal infections, sepsis remains one of the leading causes of maternal death worldwide.

Clinical features

Clinical features that suggest maternal sepsis include severe pyrexia, haemodynamic instability (tachycardia, hypotension, oliguria), tachypnoea, and impaired consciousness. However, many of these physiological parameters are already altered in the pregnant state, as described in chapter 1. Hence, a high degree of suspicion for maternal sepsis is required.

Investigations

Blood cultures must be obtained prior to initiating antibiotic therapy. If the focus of infection is not known or suspected, other samples should also be obtained (e.g. throat swabs, cerebrospinal fluid, high vaginal swab, mid-stream urine).

Serum lactate must be measured within 6 hours of sepsis being suspected. Values ≥4 mmol/L indicate tissue hypoperfusion.

Management

Intravenous broad-spectrum antibiotic coverage should begin immediately upon suspicion of maternal sepsis, after blood cultures or other samples have been collected but without waiting for microbiology results. Fluid resuscitation is required to treat hypotension and/or hypoperfusion.

Regular observation of vital signs is required, with urgent referral to the critical care team in cases of severe or rapidly deteriorating sepsis (e.g. persistent hypotension despite fluid resuscitation, respiratory failure, or significantly decreased level of consciousness).

Deep vein thrombosis and pulmonary embolism

In the postpartum period, as in pregnancy, women are at increased risk of two related conditions: deep vein thrombosis (DVT) and pulmonary embolism (referred to collectively as venous thromboembolism). In DVT, a blood clot forms in a deep vein of the lower limb and pelvis. Pulmonary embolism occurs when a part of the clot dislodges and is transported by the circulation to obstruct a blood vessel in the lungs. The embolism creates a mismatch between ventilation and perfused lung that causes shortness of breath and hypoxia. It also causes a fever and this may be the only manifestation.

Clinical features

Unilateral leg swelling, erythema and calf tenderness are signs of DVT. Pulmonary embolism is indicated by reduced oxygen saturation, chest pain and haemoptysis.

Investigations

In cases of suspected DVT, the first investigation is a Doppler US study of the affected leg and pelvic veins to look for a clot in a deep vein.

If pulmonary embolism is suspected, a chest X-ray may show opacification, meaning that the affected lung segments appear as white patches. However, the gold standard investigation for pulmonary embolism is CT pulmonary angiography (CTPA), which would show an embolus in a pulmonary artery. A ventilation-perfusion scan is another option and is associated with less radiation exposure. For this reason, VQ scan is preferred if the chest X-ray is normal as CTPA increases the lifetime risk of breast cancer by 7%, particularly in a metabolically active lactating breast. It is also the only option if there is iodinated contrast allergy or another contraindication to CTPA.

Management

The recommended treatment for both DVT and pulmonary embolism is 3–6 months of anticoagulation therapy initially with low molecular weight heparin, but subsequently with oral anticoagulation (e.g. warfarin). Urgent embolectomy is required for sizeable pulmonary emboli.

Effectiveness	Contraceptive method	Pearl index*
Low	Natural methods	3.8–20.4
	Barriers	2.5–5.9
High	Combined oral contraceptive pills	0–2.1
	Patches	0.7–1.2
	Rings	0.2–1.2
Very high	Injections	0
	Implants	0–0.3
	IUCD (copper)	0.1–1.2
	IUCD (levonorgestrel)	0–0.1
Permanent	Sterilisation	0–0.5

IUCD, intrauterine contraceptive device.
*The lower the Pearl index value, the lower the likelihood of unplanned conception.

Table 9.4 Contraception: effectiveness of different methods

9.5 Contraception and future pregnancies

It is unusual for a woman to desire pregnancy soon after giving birth, but women should have the opportunity to discuss their contraceptive options and basic contraceptive education in the postpartum period. This is also important as a short interpregnancy interval (<24 months) is associated with an increased risk of adverse outcomes in future pregnancies. The options most likely to achieve the desired contraceptive outcomes are shown in **Table 9.4**.

Index

Note: Page numbers in **bold** or *italic* refer to tables or figures respectively.

A

Abdomen, examination of 66–67, *67*
    palpation 67
    uterine size by gestational week *67*
Abdominal pain 49
    in early pregnancy **51**
    in late pregnancy **52**
    mild 49–50
    non-obstetric and non-gynaecological causes **53**
    severe 50
Abdominal palpation 198
Abdominal wall, anterior 1
    incisions *4*, 4–5
    muscles 1–3, *3*
    nerves 3
    vessels 4
Abnormal fetal condition 197
Abnormal labour 197
Abscess
    breast 228
    epidural 231
Accelerations 171
Accoucheur 81, *82*
Acute fatty liver of pregnancy (AFLP) 140, 142, 157–158
    abdominal pain in **52**
AFI *see* Amniotic fluid index (AFI)
AFLP *see* Acute fatty liver of pregnancy (AFLP)
Amniocentesis 44, *44*
Amniotic fluid index (AFI) 34–35, *35*, 72, 73
Ampicillin **126**, 155
Anaemia 62
Anaesthetic assessment, antenatal 71
Analgesia, intrapartum 85–89
    epidural anaesthesia 88
    nitrous oxide and oxygen 88
    non-pharmacological pain relief 86
    opiate injection 88–89
    perineal infiltration 87
    pharmacological pain relief 86–89
    production of pain and 86
    pudendal block 87
    spinal anaesthesia 87–88
Anencephaly *108*
Aneuploidy 101 *see also* Congenital malformations
Aneuploidy screening 32, 38–39, *40*
    types of 39, *40*
Angiotensin-converting enzyme inhibitors 162
Antenatal care 45
    abdominal pain 49–50, **51**, **52**
    breast fullness and tenderness 54
    lower back pain 52–53
    nausea and vomiting 46–49, *47*, 50–51
    peripheral oedema 54–55
    predictive and proactive model 45, *45*
    sleep disturbance 55
    trimesters of pregnancy 45, **46**
    vaginal discharge 54, **55**
Antenatal counselling 106
Antenatal visit
    first (*see* First antenatal visit)
    follow-up (*see* Follow-up antenatal visits)
Antepartum haemorrhage 131–137
    accidental causes 133, **133**
    examination 134–135
    incidental causes 131, **132**
    investigations 135, **136**
    management 135–137
    praevia causes 133, **133**
    speculum examination 135

types of morbidly adherent placenta *132*
Anti-D prophylaxis 71
Arcuate line 2, *3*
Artificial rupture of the membranes (ARM) 180–181, *182*
Assessments, in pregnancy 25
    Bishop's score 29, **29**
    engagement 27, 29
    fetal heart rate 25
    fetal lie 26, *28*
    fetal presentation 26–27
    speculum examination 29–30, *30*
    symphysis-fundal height 26, *27*
Asthma 161
Augmentation 177 *see also* Induction of labour

B

Baby blues 224
Balloon catheter insertion 180, **181**
Beckwith-Wiedemann syndrome 119
Benzodiazepine, for alcohol misuse 64
Beta-human chorionic gonadotrophin (β-hCG) 17, 50
Betamethasone 126
Biophysical profile 37–38, **39**
Birth defects *see* Congenital malformations
Bishop's score 29, **29**, 72
Bivalve speculum 30, *30*
Blood pressure, measurement of 65–66, **66**
Blood tests, antenatal 32–33
    anaemia 32
    diabetes 33
    infections, screening for 32–33
    vitamin D deficiency 32
Body mass index (BMI) 65
Booking *see* First antenatal visit
Booking-in visit *see* First antenatal visit
Braxton Hicks contractions 75–77
Breast abscess 228
Breastfeeding 221–223
    benefits of 222, **223**
    contraindications 222–223
    difficulties 219–221
    during pregnancy 54
    management **222**
    unilateral mastalgia 219
Breech presentation 71, 121–124
    external cephalic version for 122, 123
Buprenorphine, for opioid dependence 64

C

Caesarean section 194–195
    risks of **195**
Cardiac output, during pregnancy 16
Cardiotocography (CTG) 25, 30, 40–43, 72, 73, 85, 165, 197
    abnormal cardiotocograph 40, 42
    abnormal patterns **166–167**
    accelerations 171
    baseline bradycardia 167–169, *168*
    baseline tachycardia 169, *170*
    cycling 42–43
    deceleration 171–178
    Dr-C-BraVADO (mnemonic) 40, **42**
    fetal heart rate, baseline abnormal 165, 167–169
    fetal heart rate variability, abnormal patterns of 169, 171
    normal cardiotocograph 40, *41*, 42
    patterns 197
Cardiovascular disease, in pregnancy 161–162
    congenital cardiac disease 162
    ischaemic heart disease 162
Cardiovascular system, pregnancy-related changes to 14–16, *15*
    antenatal changes 15–16
    electrocardiogram in pregnancy 15
    intrapartum changes 16
    normal findings on examination 14–15
    postpartum changes 23
Carpal tunnel syndrome 54–55
Cell-free fetal DNA 39
Cervical cancer 62
Cervical insufficiency 62

Cervical ripening 177, 179–180, **180**
    balloon catheter insertion 180, **181**
    cervical membrane sweep 179
    prostaglandins 179–180, **180**
Cervical screening test 62
Childbirth, complications 197
Chorioamnionitis 124, 127, 154–155
    abdominal pain in **52**
Chorionic villus sampling (CVS) 43, *43*
Chromosomal abnormalities 101 *see also* Congenital malformations; specific type
Comfort care 106
Congenital malformations 101–107
    antenatal counselling 102
    approach to *105*
    choices to parents in 104
    Down syndrome 101, **104**
    Edwards syndrome 101, **103**
    investigations 101–103
    management of high-risk aneuploidy *106*, 106–107
    Patau syndrome 101, **102**
    Turner's syndrome 101, **105**
    ultrasound 102–104
    20-week scan 102
Conjoined twins 96
Consanguinity 63
Cord prolapse *204*, 204–205
Counselling, at first antenatal visit 68–69
CTG *see* Cardiotocography (CTG)
Cystic hygroma *107*

D

D-dimer 159
Decelerations 171–172
    early 171, *172*
    late 177, *178*
    prolonged 173, *175*, 176
    variable 173, *174*
Deep vein thrombosis 68, 233
Diabetes, in pregnancy 120–121, 149–153
    complications 150, **151**
    diagnostic approach 150–152, **152**
    gestational 150, 152–153
    insulin requirement during pregnancy 149
    pre-existing 150, 153
Diet, during pregnancy 63
Dipstick urinalysis test 145
Dizygotic twins 93, **95**, 95–96
Dopamine 18–19
Doppler assessment 35–36
    ductus venosus 36
    for fetal growth disorders 35, 109
    middle cerebral artery 36, *38*
    umbilical artery 36, *37*
    uterine artery 35, *36*
Down syndrome (trisomy 21) 39, 101, **104**
Doxylamine **156**
Ductus venosus Doppler 112, 115
Due date 60
Dysplasia 62
Dyspnoea, during pregnancy 21

E

Eclampsia 147–149
    differential diagnoses 148
    DRABC approach 148
    postpartum care 149
Ectopic pregnancy, abdominal pain in **51**
Edwards syndrome (trisomy 18) 39, 101, **103**
Endocrine system, pregnancy-related changes to 16–19, *17*, *19*
    glucose 18
    lactation 18–19
    pituitary hormones 18
    thyroid hormone levels 17, *17*
Endometritis, 228
Engagement, estimation of 27, 29
Epidural abscess 231
Episiotomy 82
Erythromycin **126**
Essential hypertension 162
Examination 64–68
    ABCD mnemonic 64–65
    abdomen 66–67, *67*
    aims of, at first antenatal visit 65

cardiovascular and respiratory systems 66
general assessment 64–65
pelvis 67–68
vital signs 65, **66**
Exercise, during pregnancy 63

F

Female reproductive system
   anterior abdominal wall 1–5, *3, 4*
   internal structures of 1, *2*
   pelvic cavity 1, *2*, 5–7
   perineum 7–8, *8, 9*
   uterus 8–9, *9*
Ferguson reflex 79
Fetal blood sampling 44
Fetal fibronectin 128
Fetal growth, disorders of 108
   asymmetrical growth 110–111
   Doppler assessment 111–115, *112–114*
   fetal biometry *109*, 109–111, *110*
   intrauterine growth restriction 115–119
   investigations 108–115
   macrosomia 119–121
   small-for-gestational-age fetus 115
Fetal growth, US assessments of 34
Fetal heart rate 67
   assessment of 25
Fetal lie 26, *28*
Fetal presentation 26–27
   breech 27
   cephalic 27
Fetal scalp lactate sampling 85
Fetoplacental circulation 10, *11*
Fetus 12
   head diameters 12, **13**, *13*
   intrapartum monitoring 85
   skull 12, *13*
   small-for-gestational-age 115
Fibroid degeneration, abdominal pain in **51**
Finger-prick blood glucose test 151
First antenatal visit 55–57
   counselling 68–69
   early in pregnancy 56
   general and obstetric examination 64–68
   history taking 56–64
   investigations **31**–**32**, 68
   lifestyle and dietary advice in 56
Folic acid supplementation 59, 68–69
Follow-up antenatal visits 69
   aim of 69
   fetal growth assessment 71
   fetal monitoring 72
   fetal presentation, assessment of 70–71
   investigations 71
   post-dates pregnancy 72–73
   questions during 69, 70
   vaginal examination and cervical membrane sweep 71
   visit schedule in uncomplicated pregnancies **70**
Forcep delivery 187
   Neville-Barnes forceps 189, *189*
   technique 192–194, *193*
   types of forceps 188–189, *189*
   Wrigley's forceps *189*

G

Gastroenteritis 229–230
Gastrointestinal changes, in pregnancy 20–21
Gastro-oesophageal reflux 163–164
Genetic disorder 62–63
Gestational age, estimation of 58, 60
Gestational diabetes 18, 63, 150, 152–153
Gestational hypertension 142–143
Glucose tolerance test 150, 152, **152**
Glycosuria 18
Graves speculum 30, *30*
Group B *Streptococcus* (GBS), screening for 72
Gynaecological history 60–62
   bleeding pattern and duration 61–62
   cervical screening 62
   irregular periods 61

menstruation 60
sexual history 62

H

Haematological changes, in pregnancy 21–22
Haematological disease 163
Haemorrhoids, during pregnancy 20
HELLP syndrome 144, 145
Hepatobiliary changes, in pregnancy 21
History taking 57–64
    age and occupation 57–58
    current pregnancy 58–59
    family history 62–63
    gynaecological history 60–62
    key aims of 57
    medical history 59
    medication history 59–60
    nutritional and physical health 63, **64**
    obstetric history 60, **61**
    rapport building and 57
    social history 63–64
    surgical history 59
Hydralazine **147**
Hyperemesis gravidarum 47, 48, 155–157
    medications **156**
    psychological support in 157
Hypertension 142, *143* *see also* Pre-eclampsia
    antihypertensive medications for 146, **146**
Hypertensive urgency 146–147, **147**
Hyperthyroidism 160–161
Hypothyroidism 160–161

I

Induction of labour 71, 72, 77, 177, 179–185
    abdominal examination 183
    artificial rupture of the membranes 180–181, *182*
    cervical ripening 177, 179–180, **180**
    indications **179**
    intrapartum care 184–185
    oxytocin infusion 181–182
    procedure for 183–185
    vaginal examination 183–184
Inferior vena cava filter 160
Inflammatory bowel disease 164
Instrumental delivery 185–194
    classification 186–187
    forceps 188–190, *189*
    FORCEPS mnemonic 185
    indications **186**
    procedure 190–194, *192, 193*
    vacuum extractor 187, **188**, *188*
Integumentary changes, in pregnancy 22–23
Intermittent auscultation (IA) 85
Intrapartum fetal monitoring 85
    cardiotocography 85
    intermittent auscultation 85
Intrauterine growth restriction (IUGR) 101, 111, 115–119, **116**, *162*
    asymmetrical 116
    delivery 119
    management 119
    risk factors **118**
    symmetrical 116
    types and causes 116, **117**
Investigations, antenatal 30, **31–32**
    amniocentesis 44, *44*
    aneuploidy screening 38–39, *40*
    blood tests 32–33
    cardiotocography 40–43, *41*, **42**
    chorionic villus sampling 43, *43*
    fetal blood sampling 44
    imaging 33–38
    urine tests 33
Iodine, in pregnancy 59
Iron-deficiency anaemia 163
IUGR *see* Intrauterine growth restriction (IUGR)

J

Joel-Cohen incision 4

K

Kleihauer–Betke test 128

L

Labetalol **146, 147**
Labour 75 *see also* Induction of labour
    abdominal pain in **52**
    cardinal movements of *81–82*
    cord clamping 82–84
    dystocia 197
    first stage 77–79, *78*
    intrapartum analgesia 85–89
    intrapartum monitoring 85
    latent phase 75–77
    monitoring during 75
    peripartum and intrapartum cervical change 76
    progress of normal labour *78*
    rule of three 75
    second stage 79–84
    stages of **77**
    stations of fetal descent *83*, 84
    third stage 84
    three P's 6
    vaginal examinations 78, 79
Lactation 18–19, *19*
Laparoscopy incision 5
Last menstrual period (LMP) 60, 61
Leopold's manoeuvres 26, *28*
Levator ani 7–8, *8*
Levothyroxine 161
Lidocaine 87
Liver disease, in pregnancy 139–142
    causes **141**
Lower back pain 52–53

M

Macrosomia 119–121
Magnesium sulphate, for eclamptic seizure 148, 149
Malpresentation 121 *see also* Breech presentation
    caesarean section 124
    external cephalic version 122, *123*
    planned vaginal breech birth 124
    types of 121, *122*
Mask of pregnancy 22
Mastitis 226–227

Maternal age 58
Maternal sepsis 232–233
Maternity record 48
Medication history 59–60
Melasma 22
Meningomyelocele 108
Metformin, in pregnancy 152
Methyldopa **146**
Metoclopramide **156**
Middle cerebral artery Doppler 112, *114*
Midline incisions 5
Midwife 56
Mini-Mental State Examination 220
Miscarriage, abdominal pain in **51**
Model of care 56
Monozygotic twins 93, 95, **95**
Multiparous uterus 182
Multiple pregnancy 91–93 *see also* Twin pregnancy
Multivitamin **156**
Musculoskeletal changes, in pregnancy 22

N

Naegele's rule, for estimated date of birth 61
Nausea and vomiting 46–49, 50–51
    differential diagnoses **47**
Neural tube defects 108
Nifedipine **126, 146**
Non-cephalic presentation *see* Malpresentation
Nuchal thickness
    increased *107*
    normal *107*

O

Obstetric examinations 64 *see also* Examination
Obstetrician 56
Ondansetron **156**
Ovarian hyperstimulation syndrome, abdominal pain in **51**
Ovarian torsion, abdominal pain in **51**
Oxytocin infusion 181–182

P

Papanicolaou's test 62
Parasitic twins 96
Patau syndrome (trisomy 13) 39, 101, **102**
Pederson speculum 30
Pelvic floor 7, 79
Pelvis 5
    dimensions 6–7
    examination of 67–68
    greater bony pelvis 6
    lesser bony pelvis 5–6, *6*
Peptic ulcer disease 163–164
Perinatal depression 224–225
Perineal infiltration 87
Perineal tears, during childbirth 7
Perineum
    anatomy of *7*–8, *8*
    urogenital and anal triangles of 8, *9*
Peripheral oedema 54–55
Pfannenstiel incision 4, *4*
Physiological changes, in pregnancy 13–14, 45
    cardiovascular changes 14–16, *15*
    endocrine changes 16–19, *17*, *19*
    gastrointestinal changes 20–21
    haematological changes 21–22
    immunological changes 23
    integumentary changes 22–23
    musculoskeletal changes 22
    normal values of physiological variables in pregnancy **14**
    respiratory changes 21, *22*
    urological changes 19–20
Physiological third stage 84
Pinard's manoeuvre 198
Placenta 9
    changes after birth 10
    decidua 10
    early development and structure 10
    fetoplacental circulation 10, *11*
    function of 9–10
Placenta accreta *132*, 134
Placenta increta *132*
Placental abruption, abdominal pain in **52**
Placenta percreta *132*
Placenta praevia 134
Pneumonia 230–231
    risk factors **227**
Polycystic ovarian syndrome 61
Polycythaemia 100
Post-dates pregnancy 72–73
Postpartum haemorrhage (PPH) 84, 182, 210–217
    causes **212**
    classification 211–212
    follow-up care for *216*
    management 212
    medications **213**
Postpartum pyrexia 226
Post-term pregnancy *see* Post-dates pregnancy
PPROM *see* Preterm prelabour rupture of membranes (PPROM)
Prednisolone **156**
Pre-eclampsia 142–145, *143*
    abdominal pain in **52**
    defined 143
    hypertension and 65, 142
    screening for 60, 63
    severe 144–145
Pregnancy
    biological factor 223
    emotional factor 223
    gravidity and parity 60, 61
    multivitamins 59
    social factor 224
Prelabour rupture of membranes 79
Prenatal development 11
    embryonic phase 11–12
    fetal phase 12
    stages of **12**
Presentation 121 *see also* Malpresentation
Preterm labour 127–131
    delivery 130
    fetal fibronectin test 128
    medications for management in 129, **129**
    prognosis *130*, 130–131
    twin pregnancy 98

Preterm prelabour rupture of
  membranes (PPROM) 124–127
    delivery 127
    medications for management 126,
      126
Primigravid uterus 182
Prochlorperazine **156**
Promethazine **156**
Prostaglandins, for cervical ripening
  179–180, **180**
Proteinuria 142, 145
Psychiatric illness 224
Pudendal block 87
Pulmonary embolism 158–160, 233
Pulmonary oedema, in pregnancy 16
Pyelonephritis 229
Pushing 81
Pyelonephritis 20, 33
Pyramidalis muscle 2–3
Pyridoxine (vitamin B6) **156**

Q
Quadruplets 93
Quickening 69

R
Ranitidine **156**
Rectus abdominis 1–2, *3*
Relaxin 22
Renal disease, in pregnancy 162–163
Respiratory changes, in pregnancy 21,
  22
Respiratory disease 161
Respiratory distress syndrome 130
Retained products of conception 10
Ruptured ovarian cyst, abdominal pain
  in **51**

S
Sciatica 53
Sexually transmitted infections 62
Sheehan's syndrome 18
Shoulder dystocia 120, 205–208, *206*
  management of 207–208
  risk factors **207**
Shouldering 173

Show 54, 69, 75
Sickle cell disease 163
Sleep disturbance, during pregnancy 55
Small-for-gestational-age (SGA) fetus
  115
Speculum examination 29–30, *30*
Spinal anaesthesia 87–88
Stretch marks 22–23
Substance misuse, in pregnancy 63–64
Suckling 18–19
Surgical history 59
Symphysis-fundal height 26, *27*, 67,
  108

T
Terbutaline 176
Thalassaemia 163
Thiamine (vitamin B1) supplementation
  64, 155, **156**
Thyroid dysfunction, during pregnancy
  160–161
Thyroid function test 220
Thyroid-stimulating hormone (TSH) 17
Triplets 93
TTTS *see* Twin-to-twin transfusion
  syndrome (TTTS)
Turner's syndrome 101, **105**
Twin anaemia polycythaemia sequence
  100–101
Twin pregnancy 93
  amnionicity 94, **94**
  chorionicity 93, **94**, 96
  conjoined twins 96
  descriptive terms for **94**
  dizygotic twins **95**, 95–96
  fetal complications, risk of 97–98,
    98
  maternal complications, risk of **97**,
    97–98
  monozygotic twins 95, **95**
  parasitic twins 96
  preterm labour 98
  T sign 96
  twin anaemia polycythaemia
    sequence 100–101
  twin reversed arterial perfusion 96

twin-to-twin transfusion syndrome 98–100, **99**
zygosity 93, **94**
Twin reversed arterial perfusion (TRAP) 96
Twin-to-twin transfusion syndrome (TTTS) 98–100
    fetal outcomes 100
    Quintero's stage **99**
Type 1 diabetes mellitus 150

U

Ultrasound, antenatal 33–38, 61, 72, 96
    advantages 34
    amniotic fluid index 34–35, *35*
    biophysical profile 37–38, **39**
    congenital malformations 102–104
    Doppler assessment 35–36, *36, 37, 38*
    indications 33–34
    US dating scan 34
Umbilical arteries 10, *11*
Umbilical artery Doppler 111–113
    absent end-diastolic flow *113*
    decrease in diastolic flow *113*
    reversed end-diastolic flow *114*
    systolic to diastolic flow (SD ratio) *113*
Umbilical cord 10
    clamping 82–84
Umbilical vein 10, *11*
Unilateral mastalgia 219
Urinary stasis 20
Urinary tract infections 229
Urinary urgency 20
Urine tests 33
Urological changes, in pregnancy 19–20
    bladder function 20
    renal function 20
Uterine artery Doppler 111, *112*
Uterine inversion 208–210, *209*
Uterine rupture, abdominal pain in **52**
Uterotonic agent/oxytocic 83
Uterus 8
    anatomy of 8, *9*
    blood supply to 9
    relations of 8

V

Vacuum-assisted delivery 187, *188*
    advantages and disadvantages **188**
    technique 191–192, *192*
Vaginal breech birth
    contraindication 199
    fetal injury 200–201
    risks 199
Vaginal discharge 54
    show 54
    types indicating infection **55**
    watery 54
Vanishing twin syndrome 97
Varicose veins 68
Venous thromboembolism 158–160
Virchow's triad 158
Vitamin D, in pregnancy 59

W

Warm compresses 81
Weight gain, recommended, in pregnancy **64**
Wernicke's encephalopathy 155
Womb mates 95

Z

Zero station *83*, 84